Family Sleep Solutions
A Guide to Restful Nights

Unlocking the Secrets of Sleep Health for Children and Adults through Breathing Exercises, Meditation, and Practical Strategies

Jasper Blich

COPYRIGHT © 2023

Notice of Copyright

All rights reserved.

No part of this publication may be reproduced, stored in a retrieval system, stored in a database, and / or published in any form or by any means, electronic, mechanical, photocopying, recording, or otherwise, without the prior written permission of the publisher.

Written by: Jasper Blich

TABLE OF CONTENTS

TABLE OF CONTENTS

INTRODUCTION

Why Sleep Matters for Parents and Kids

Common Sleep Problems

Objectives of this Book

1.   UNDERSTANDING SLEEP

Sleep Cycles Explained
  NREM Stage 1 (Light Sleep)
  NREM Stage 2 (Moderate Sleep)
  NREM Stage 3 (Deep Sleep)
  REM Sleep (Rapid Eye Movement Sleep)

The Sleep Needs of Adults
  Sleep Duration
  Sleep Quality
  Impact of Lifestyle Choices
  Importance of Sleep for Cognitive Functions
  Sleep Disorders in Adults

The Sleep Needs of Children
  Sleep Duration by Age
  Importance of Quality Sleep
  Sleep Environment and Routine
  Effects of Sleep Deprivation
  Addressing Sleep Problems
  Role of Parents and Caregivers

Identifying Sleep Problems
  Common Sleep Problems

Recognizing Symptoms
Role of Sleep Diary
Effects of Sleep Problems
Consulting a Professional
Treatment Options
Prevention and Early Intervention

2.   PREPARING FOR BETTER SLEEP

Importance of Sleep Environment
Understanding Sleep Environment
Lighting
Temperature
Noise Level
Comfort of Bedding
Cleanliness and Organization
Aromatherapy
Electronics-Free Zone
Personalized Touches
Importance for Children

Tips for Adults
Establish a Routine
Limit Exposure to Screens Before Bedtime
Mindful Eating and Drinking
Create a Bedtime Ritual
Exercise Regularly but Not Too Late in the Day
Manage Stress
Optimize the Sleep Environment
Be Mindful of Naps
Seek Professional Help if Needed
Consider the Needs of Others

Tips for Children
Establish a Consistent Sleep Schedule
Create a Calming Bedtime Routine
Optimize the Sleep Environment
Avoid Screen Time Before Bed
Encourage Physical Activity
Be Mindful of Food and Drink
Provide a Comfort Item if Needed
Communicate About Sleep
Limit Naps for Older Children
Respond to Nighttime Waking Calmly
Seek Professional Help if Needed

Special Considerations for Children with Special Needs
Understanding the Specific Needs
Develop a Tailored Sleep Routine

Create a Sensory-Friendly Environment
Consider Medication and Dietary Factors
Utilize Adaptive Equipment if Necessary
Provide Clear Communication
Focus on Emotional Support
Monitor Sleep Patterns
Engage in Collaborative Care
Educate Siblings and Other Family Members
Consider Professional Sleep Consultation

3. INTRODUCTION TO BREATHING EXERCISES

What Are Breathing Exercises?
Connection to Mind-Body Practices
Different Types of Breathing Exercises
Integrating Breathing Exercises into Sleep Routines

Benefits of Breathing Exercises
Stress Reduction
Improvement in Sleep Quality
Enhanced Emotional Well-being
Support for Respiratory Health
Cardiovascular Health Benefits
Pain Management
Enhanced Concentration and Focus
Support for Digestive Health
Complementary to Other Therapies

Getting Started with Breathing Exercises
Understanding the Purpose
Find a Comfortable Space
Adopt a Comfortable Position
Start with Simple Techniques
Focus on Quality, Not Quantity
Use Technology If Needed
Consistency is Key
Monitor Your Progress
Explore Different Techniques
Consult Professionals if Necessary

Breathing Exercises to Improve Sleep
Progressive Relaxation
The 4-7-8 Method
Diaphragmatic Breathing (Belly Breathing)
Guided Meditation and Visualization
Humming Bee Breath (Bhramari Pranayama)
Box Breathing

4. BREATHING EXERCISES FOR FAMILIES

Why Practice with Your Kids?
Bonding and Connection
Emotional Regulation
Stress Reduction
Enhancing Focus and Concentration
Encouraging Healthy Habits
Adaptation and Customization
Improving Sleep Patterns
Building Empathy and Understanding

Exercises You Can Do Together
Balloon Breaths
Animal Breaths
Counting Breaths
Partner Breathing
Guided Relaxation

Tips for Success
Start Slow
Make it a Routine
Use Props and Visuals
Be Patient and Supportive
Modify as Needed
Lead by Example
Focus on Enjoyment
Communicate Openly
Monitor Progress

Tracking Progress Together
Why Monitor Progress?
Methods for Tracking Progress
Considerations and Tips

5. INTRODUCTION TO MEDITATION

What Is Meditation?
Historical Background
Types of Meditation
Purposes and Goals
How to Get Started

How to Get Started with Meditation
Selecting the Right Technique
Finding Guidance
Setting Up Your Space
Determining the Duration

Developing a Routine
Practicing Mindfully
Tracking Progress
Seeking Community

Meditation Techniques for Better Sleep
Guided Sleep Meditation
Progressive Muscle Relaxation
Mindfulness Meditation
Deep Breathing Techniques
Yoga Nidra (Yogic Sleep)
Visualization Techniques
Mantra Meditation
Incorporating Sleep-Inducing Sounds

Meditation Techniques You Can Do with Your Kids
Animal Breathing Meditation
Story Meditation
Mindful Coloring or Drawing
Bubble Breathing Exercise
The Gratitude Meditation
Guided Imagery with Stuffed Animals
The Sound Game
Body Scanning with a Toy
Flower and Candle Breathing
Partner Yoga and Meditation

6. ENHANCING SLEEP THROUGH MEDITATION

How Meditation Improves Sleep
Calming the Mind
Reducing Stress Hormones
Enhancing Relaxation
Regulating the Sleep-Wake Cycle
Improving Sleep Quality
Addressing Specific Sleep Disorders
Fostering a Bedtime Ritual
Promoting Emotional Well-Being

Implementing Meditation into Your Routine
Start Small
Find the Right Time and Place
Use Guided Meditations
Create a Meditation Space
Be Consistent
Involve Your Family
Experiment with Different Techniques
Combine Meditation with Other Activities
Keep a Meditation Journal

Be Patient and Kind to Yourself
Seek Support if Needed

Guiding Children Through Meditation
Understand Their Needs and Interests
Start with Short Sessions
Create a Calming Environment
Use Simple Techniques
Incorporate Imagery and Storytelling
Be Patient and Positive
Include Movement
Emphasize Sensory Experience
Provide Reassurance and Guidance
Make It a Regular Practice
Celebrate Progress
Include Them in Your Practice

Measuring Improvements in Sleep
Keep a Sleep Journal
Use Technology
Observe Changes in Daytime Functioning
Monitor Physical Health Indicators
Assess Children's Sleep Through Communication
Look for a Reduction in Sleep Problems
Consider Professional Assessment if Needed
Focus on Consistency
Reflect on the Impact of Implemented Techniques
Involve Children in the Process

7. STRATEGIES FOR SPECIAL NEEDS CHILDREN

Understanding Specific Needs (e.g., ADHD)
ADHD and Sleep Challenges
Understanding Other Specific Needs
Tailored Strategies for Specific Needs
Using Medication Thoughtfully

Tailored Strategies for Better Sleep
Assessing Individual Needs
Creating a Supportive Sleep Environment
Establishing Consistent Bedtime Routines
Using Technology and Tools
Incorporating Behavioral Strategies
Educating and Involving the Family
Ongoing Evaluation and Adjustment

Supporting Parents and Caregivers
Providing Education and Training
Creating Support Systems

Offering Emotional Support
Access to Professional Guidance
Providing Practical Tools and Resources
Encouraging Self-Care
Fostering a Collaborative Approach

Resources and Support
Educational Resources
Professional Support
Community Support
Technology and Tools
Government and Non-Profit Organizations
Schools and Educational Institutions

8. IMPROVING SLEEP FOR ADULTS

Assessing Your Sleep Quality
Understanding the Importance of Sleep Quality
Identifying Signs of Poor Sleep Quality
Utilizing Sleep Assessment Tools
Reflecting on Lifestyle and Environmental Factors

Strategies for Improvement
Creating a Consistent Sleep Routine
Mindful Eating and Drinking
Managing Stress and Anxiety
Seek Professional Help if Needed
Avoiding Substance Abuse
Understanding Individual Needs

How Meditation and Breathing Intertwine
The Foundation of Awareness
Calming the Mind and Body
Enhancing Sleep Quality
Personalized Approach
Holistic Health Benefits

Common Pitfalls and How to Avoid Them
Expecting Immediate Results
Lack of Consistency
Choosing Inappropriate Techniques
Ignoring Underlying Issues
Overemphasis on One Approach
Pressuring Yourself
Ignoring the Needs of Children (if applicable)

9. IMPROVING SLEEP FOR CHILDREN

Assessing Your Child's Sleep Quality

Understanding Sleep Needs by Age
Observing Sleep Patterns and Behavior
Using a Sleep Diary or Journal
Considering Environmental Factors
Consulting with Professionals if Needed

Strategies for Improvement
Establish a Consistent Sleep Schedule
Create a Relaxing Bedtime Routine
Ensure a Comfortable Sleep Environment
Encourage Healthy Sleep Habits
Teach Self-Soothing Techniques
Communicate and Collaborate
Consider Professional Assistance if Needed

Teaching Kids About Sleep Health
Start with the Basics: What Is Sleep and Why Do We Need It?
Introduce the Concept of a Sleep Routine
Talk About Good Sleep Hygiene
Discuss Different Sleep Stages
Teach Them to Recognize Sleepiness Signs
Promote the Connection Between Sleep and Health
Utilize Interactive Learning Tools
Reinforce and Review

Overcoming Common Challenges
Bedtime Resistance
Nightmares and Night Terrors
Sleep Anxiety
Sleepwalking
Screen Time Before Bed
Inconsistent Sleep Schedules
Snoring and Breathing Issues

10. BRINGING IT ALL TOGETHER

How Breathing and Meditation Work Together
Connection to the Present Moment
Breath as a Tool
Building Awareness
Calming the Mind
Synergistic Effects
Holistic Approach
Enhancing Sleep Quality
Integrated Practice

Creating a Family Sleep Routine
Assess Individual Needs
Incorporate Personalization

Establish Consistency
Set a Schedule
Create a Supportive Environment
Minimize Distractions
Include Soothing Elements
Incorporate Family Participation
Family Bonding Time
Modeling Healthy Habits

Monitoring Progress and Making Adjustments
Keeping Track
Review and Analyze
Make Necessary Adjustments
Celebrate Progress

Final Words of Encouragement
Embrace the Journey
Family Connection
Focus on Well-Being
Stay Positive
Keep Exploring
You've Got This

SUMMARY

INTRODUCTION

Sleep is a vital biological function that significantly affects general health and well-being. Sleep is essential for many physiological and neurological processes; it does more than merely allow the body to rest.

The brain cycles through various stages of sleep while we are unconscious, including REM (Rapid Eye Movement) and non-REM sleep. There are three stages of non-REM sleep, each of which contributes differently to the body's recovery. Slow-wave sleep, often referred to as deep sleep, is especially important for memory consolidation and physical healing.

These cycles are controlled by the circadian rhythm, or internal body clock, which synchronizes our sleep cycles with the 24-hour day. Sleep issues can result from any disturbances to this routine, such as shift work or traveling between time zones.

Why Sleep Matters for Parents and Kids

Although sleep is necessary for both adults and children, its functions vary depending on the stage of life. Adults who get enough sleep are better able to operate cognitively, have stable moods, and stay physically healthy. It interferes with our capacity for clear thinking, decision-making, and even social interaction.

On the other hand, because their bodies and brains are still growing and developing, children need more sleep. In children, sleep fosters development, aids learning, improves mood, and strengthens the immune system. Children who do not receive sufficient sleep may have behavioral problems, academic difficulties, or health issues.

The ability of parents to care for their children, handle everyday tasks, and keep a happy home atmosphere depends on how well they sleep. Sleep is not just a personal matter, it can also impact the dynamics of the entire family.

Common Sleep Problems

Sleep issues can affect both adults and children and can take on different forms. These may consist of:

Insomnia, is the inability to get to sleep or stay asleep.
Sleep apnea is a disorder characterized by repeated pauses in breathing while sleeping.
The Restless Legs Syndrome is characterized by an unpleasant feeling in the legs that causes an overwhelming need to move.
Nightmares and night terrors are particularly prevalent in young children.
Circadian Rhythm Disorders cause the internal body clock to be out of sync.

These problems have the potential to greatly affect one's physical health, mental well-being, and overall quality of life. They could also be a sign of underlying medical problems.

Objectives of this Book

This book's main goal is to give parents and kids useful, tested strategies for improving the quality of their sleep through breathing and meditation. It attempts to investigate the connection between breathing, meditation, and sleep while providing knowledge and strategies for resolving typical sleep issues.

The book will also act as a thorough instruction manual, covering not just the techniques but also the underlying science, advantages, and applicability for various age groups and particular needs. It will provide readers the capacity to control their sleep, cultivate better habits, and have a beneficial knock-on effect on their lives as a whole.

1. UNDERSTANDING SLEEP

Our daily lives depend on sleep, which is essential to preserving our physical and mental well-being. Our bodies go through various sleep cycles when we sleep, which are crucial for self-restoration and renewal. Rapid Eye Movement (REM) sleep and Non-Rapid Eye Movement (NREM) sleep are the two primary categories of sleep cycles.

Sleep Cycles Explained

The concept of sleep cycles is essential to comprehending both how we sleep and the processes that take place while we are dozing off. During the night, our brain and body progress through a series of distinct stages, each of which is associated with a distinct set of features and alterations in our physiology.

NREM Stage 1 (Light Sleep)

NREM, the first stage of sleep, often known as the stage of light sleep, is characterized by a transition from waking to sleep. It is a time during which a person can be readily roused from sleep. The time allotted for this stage is somewhere between one and five minutes. A decrease in heart rate and a loosening up of the muscles are two examples of the physiological changes that take place. This stage is the beginning of the sleep cycle and it is often accompanied by the feeling of falling. It also marks the beginning of the sleep cycle.

NREM Stage 2 (Moderate Sleep)

After a period of light sleep, an individual will go on to NREM

Stage 2, which is characterized by more moderate levels of sleep. This stage lasts for anything between ten and twenty-five minutes, on average. During this stage, the temperature of the body declines, the heart rate continues to slow down, and ocular movements completely stop. This stage is distinguished by the presence of sleep spindles, which are brief periods of heightened brain activity.

NREM Stage 3 (Deep Sleep)

NREM, or deep sleep is the third stage of the sleep cycle and is known as the most restorative stage. It can last anywhere between 20 and 40 minutes. During this phase, the body will work to mend damaged tissues, develop new bone and muscle, and fortify the immune system. Growth hormones are only released when a person is in a deep sleep stage. This stage is essential for both the physical well-being of the body and its recuperation from the activities of daily life.

REM Sleep (Rapid Eye Movement Sleep)

REM sleep, also known as rapid eye movement sleep, is the stage of sleep in which individuals experience increased brain activity, fast eye movements, and dreaming. The initial cycle of REM sleep typically lasts between 10 and 20 minutes, but the duration of REM sleep in the following cycles grows longer. REM sleep typically begins about 90 minutes after falling asleep. This stage is extremely important for both the consolidation of memories and the learning process.

The complexity of sleep, as well as the ways in which different stages of sleep contribute to overall health and well-being, can be better understood by having a better grasp of these cycles. It demonstrates why getting enough quality sleep is more important than getting enough amount of sleep, given that distinct stages of sleep each fulfill a different set of necessary duties. One can begin to comprehend the significant part that sleep plays in both day-to-day life and general wellness once they have gained an understanding of the nature of these cycles.

The Sleep Needs of Adults

It is essential for adults, whose ages typically range from 18 to 64 years old, to meet certain sleep requirements in order to preserve their overall health, mental well-being, and everyday performance. By gaining an understanding of these requirements, individuals can be guided in prioritizing their sleep habits, resulting in a life that is more balanced and productive.

Sleep Duration

The average amount of sleep that an adult should get each night is between seven and nine hours. Sleep deprivation, which can cause mood changes, memory problems, and difficulty concentrating, might be the result of getting fewer than this amount of hours in bed each night. On the other hand, sleeping for significantly longer than the amount of time that is suggested can be an indicator of underlying health problems or poor sleep quality.

Sleep Quality

The caliber of one's slumber is just as important as the total amount that one gets. A pleasant resting environment, a regular sleep schedule, and the avoidance of interruptions such as loud noises and bright lights are all factors that contribute to good sleep quality. Adults need to have sleep cycles that are both lengthy and uninterrupted if they want to feel ready to face the demands of the next day when they wake up.

Impact of Lifestyle Choices

Adults' needs for sleep are strongly impacted by the decisions they make regarding their lifestyle. Consuming alcohol, caffeine, or large meals in the hours leading up to night can reduce the quality of sleep you get. Better sleep can be promoted by engaging in regular physical activity, maintaining a healthy diet, and using stress management techniques. In addition, avoiding the use of electronic gadgets before going to bed, such as cellphones and laptops, might send a message to the brain that it is time to relax and wind down.

Importance of Sleep for Cognitive Functions

Memory, decision-making, creativity, and critical thinking are all cognitive processes that benefit greatly from getting enough quality sleep. The capacity of the brain to establish connections between disparate pieces of information is improved during sleep, which in turn supports creative and original thought. These cognitive functions can be hindered by a lack of enough sleep, which can result in a reduction in one's ability to be productive at work and to solve problems.

Sleep Disorders in Adults

Sleep disorders such as insomnia, sleep apnea, and restless leg syndrome affect a significant number of adult patients nowadays. If not treated, these conditions can cause a disruption in the natural cycle of sleep, which in turn can result in chronic sleep deprivation. It is essential to get a proper diagnosis and treatment to restore good sleep patterns. Treatment typically consists of a combination of medication, therapy, and changes in lifestyle.

Adults have complex sleep requirements that are shaped by a variety of circumstances, including their age, lifestyle, health issues, and individual routines and routines. Understanding and satisfying these requirements can lead to improvements in one's physical health, mental acuity, and overall life happiness. Both the quality and quantity of the requirements should be given equal weight. It is not enough to simply get the recommended amount of sleep; rather, one must make sleep a priority and acknowledge the critical function that sleep plays in each and every facet of daily life.

The Sleep Needs of Children

The amount of sleep that is necessary for children varies greatly according to their age; however, sleep is extremely important to a child's general physical development, emotional maturity, intellectual progress, and sense of well-being. A more in-depth look at these prerequisites is as follows:

Sleep Duration by Age

Infants (0-3 months)

14–17 hours a day on average. Their slumber is fragmented throughout the day and night, and the rhythms of their sleeping are determined by their requirements for food.

Babies (4-11 months)

12–15 hours a day on average. The usual sleep pattern returns, and they establish a more reliable routine for when they go to bed each night.

Toddlers (1-2 years)

11-14 hours a day on average. They begin to incorporate catnaps into their daily routine, which results in increased time spent asleep during the night.

Preschoolers (3-5 years)

10–13 hours a day on average. Your napping habits may change, but you'll end up sleeping through the night more consistently.

School-age Children (6-13 years)

9-11 hours per night on average. It is crucial for this age group to have a regular schedule for going to bed to guarantee that they get enough rest.

Importance of Quality Sleep

Children's mental and physical development are both significantly impacted by the quality of sleep they get, making it essential for them to get enough of it. The release of growth hormones, which are necessary for normal, healthy growth, occurs during deep sleep. Remembering things more clearly, being more creative, and developing better social skills are all aided by getting enough quality sleep.

Sleep Environment and Routine

Better sleep can be encouraged in children by establishing a regular bedtime routine as well as a relaxing atmosphere in which they sleep. The right environment for sleep can be created with the help of low lighting, soothing music, and reassuring stories before bed. The child's internal body clock can be more easily synchronized if the child keeps to a consistent sleep routine even on the weekends.

Effects of Sleep Deprivation

Children who do not get enough sleep are more likely to display behavioral concerns, have mood swings, struggle academically, and develop health problems such as obesity. Sleep deprivation, especially if it's chronic, can potentially cause long-term problems with cognition and emotion.

Addressing Sleep Problems

Children frequently have a variety of sleep issues, including recurring nightmares, sleepwalking, and trouble falling or staying asleep. These concerns must be recognized by parents and other caregivers, and if necessary, professional assistance must be sought out to address them. Changing the environment in which you sleep, establishing a pattern for going to bed, or addressing the underlying fears that may be keeping you up at night are all potential strategies.

Role of Parents and Caregivers

When it comes to identifying and meeting the sleeping requirements of their children, parents, and other caretakers play a vital role. Parents can instill in their children healthy sleeping routines that will be to their children's benefit for the rest of their lives if they pay attention to these demands and create an environment that is conducive to sleep.

Children have complicated sleep requirements, and those requirements change at each stage of their development. These requirements must be met to support their development, learning, emotional well-being, and overall health. By understanding these demands and making sleep a priority, parents may lay the groundwork for their child's lifetime health and well-being, fostering not only the child's physical development but also their mental and spiritual growth.

Identifying Sleep Problems

For both adults and kids, discovering sleep issues can be a serious worry. The first step in resolving these problems is proper identification of them.

Common Sleep Problems

Insomnia

Even under ideal circumstances, it is characterized by difficulty falling or staying asleep. It may be a recurring problem or only happens rarely.

Sleep Apnea

A potentially life-threatening sleep disorder characterized by frequent pauses and restarts of breathing. Snoring and daytime weariness could result from it.

Restless Leg Syndrome (RLS)

Having the painful impulse to move one's legs, especially during the night, might make it difficult to sleep.

Narcolepsy

A persistent sleep condition that is characterized by extreme daytime sleepiness and unexpected bouts of sleep during the day.

Nightmares and Night Terrors

They are especially prevalent in youngsters and can cause disturbed sleep as well as a fear of sleeping.

Recognizing Symptoms

Observing sleep patterns and daytime behavior is necessary to spot sleep issues. These symptoms could point to a sleep disorder:

Frequent Wakefulness

Having several awakenings throughout the night.

Daytime Fatigue

Having persistent feelings of exhaustion or falling asleep during the daytime.

Changes in Behavior

Mood fluctuations, impatience, and an inability to concentrate are all symptoms of this condition.

Physical Symptoms

Snoring, gasping for breath while sleeping, and restless legs are all signs of sleep-disordered breathing.

Role of Sleep Diary

Keeping a sleep journal can be a helpful tool for figuring out sleep issues. Recording your bedtime, wake-up time, overall sleep duration, interruptions, and morning moods might help you spot patterns or abnormalities that could indicate a specific problem.

Effects of Sleep Problems

Physical health problems including heart disease, obesity, diabetes, and even a compromised immune system can develop as a result of untreated sleep difficulties. Additionally, mental health issues like sadness, anxiety, and cognitive decline might result.

Consulting a Professional

It could be necessary to speak with a healthcare professional if self-monitoring and modifications to sleep hygiene are ineffective at solving the issues. They can do a full evaluation and can even suggest a sleep study at a dedicated sleep facility.

Treatment Options

Depending on the kind and severity of the condition, many treatments are available for sleep disorders. In the case of problems like sleep apnea, it may also involve medical equipment, therapy, medicine, or lifestyle modifications.

Prevention and Early Intervention

Knowing the value of sleep and spotting the early warning

signals of sleep difficulties can help prompt care and avert more serious health problems. Sleep-related problems can often be avoided with the help of consistent sleep schedules, a comfortable sleeping environment, and awareness of personal sleep requirements.

Finding solutions to sleep issues is essential for overall health. It entails identifying symptoms, comprehending their effects, and, if necessary, obtaining expert assistance. The quality of life can be improved with prompt intervention and appropriate care, which will have a favorable impact on all facets of everyday life. To identify these issues early and take the necessary steps to restore healthy sleep patterns, awareness, and education are essential.

2.
PREPARING FOR BETTER SLEEP

To sleep well, an appropriate sleeping environment must be created. The environment that you sleep in includes things like light, noise, temperature, humidity, and comfort. A comfortable sleeping environment can encourage unwinding, lessen stress, and enhance the general effectiveness of sleep.

Importance of Sleep Environment

The setting in which we sleep has a big impact on how well we sleep. Lighting, temperature, noise, and the surrounding environment can all help or hinder getting a good night's sleep. Let's go specifically about setting up the best environment for sleeping.

Understanding Sleep Environment

The physical circumstances in which one sleeps are referred to as the sleep environment. It covers everything from the bed and pillows to the bedding arrangement, furniture, lighting, temperature, and noise level in the bedroom.

Lighting

For sleeping, soft, dark illumination is preferred. The hormone that promotes sleep, melatonin, can be inhibited by exposure to bright lights before bed. A relaxing effect can be produced by using nightlights or dimmable lighting.

Temperature

The temperature of the bedroom has a big impact on how well you sleep. Better sleep is encouraged by a somewhat chilly bedroom, usually between 60- and 67 degrees Fahrenheit (15 to 19 degrees Celsius). The room temperature should be set to coincide with the body's natural cooling process as it gets ready for sleep to promote restful sleep.

Noise Level

A peaceful setting is necessary for uninterrupted sleep. White noise generators or relaxing background music can help block out outdoor noise and create a relaxing environment.

Comfort of Bedding

It can be quite beneficial to spend money on a comfy mattress, pillows, and bedding that meet personal preferences. Personal comfort requirements should be taken into account while choosing the stiffness, height, and texture of the pillow and mattress.

Cleanliness and Organization

A space that is tidy and free of clutter has a calming effect. Unconsciously, the disorder can lead to more tension, which can make it difficult to sleep.

Aromatherapy

Relaxation can be encouraged by some smells, such as lavender. Diffusers for essential oils or scented candles can provide an extra layer of comfort.

Electronics-Free Zone

Blue light from screens can interfere with the body's natural cycle of sleep and wakefulness. Keeping electronics like phones, iPads, and televisions out of the bedroom can make it easier to fall asleep.

Personalized Touches

It is possible to create a more pleasant sleeping environment by incorporating special touches that promote peace and relaxation. It might contain souvenirs, artwork, or your favorite colors.

Importance for Children

Children also need a conducive sleeping environment, especially newborns and toddlers. It is easier for kids to adapt to sleep when the environment where they sleep is consistent and associated with bedtime.

The environment in which you sleep affects the quality of your sleep in more ways than one. Customizing the sleeping environment to meet unique needs and tastes is not a luxury, but rather a requirement for sound sleep. Every component, from the lighting to the bedding, should be carefully picked to create a sanctuary that promotes relaxation and renewal. A restorative night's sleep that enhances general well-being is fostered by this attentive approach to the sleep environment, which creates the right conditions for the body and mind to unwind. It's a move that embodies self-care in its purest form and leads the road to better everyday performance and life quality.

Tips for Adults

When it comes to getting a good night's sleep, adults frequently confront a unique set of obstacles. Several things can get in the way of getting quality sleep, including stress from work, the demands of family life, and the difficulty of balancing one's personal and professional lives. An insightful guide on practical sleep tips that are geared specifically toward adults is presented here.

Establish a Routine

The body's internal clock can be trained with the use of a routine. Maintaining a regular bedtime and rising at the same time each day can help to normalize the sleep-wake cycle that occurs naturally in the body. The weekends should not be treated differently because significant deviations from this routine can throw it off.

Limit Exposure to Screens Before Bedtime

Melatonin production is inhibited by the blue light that is emitted by electronic devices like cellphones, tablets, and computers. If you want to assist your mind wind down and send a signal to your body that it's time to rest, avoiding screens for at least an hour before bed is a good idea.

Mindful Eating and Drinking

Consuming large meals, beverages containing caffeine, or alcohol too soon tonight might disrupt sleep. A better night's sleep can be facilitated by choosing a food that is lower in calories, avoiding caffeine after the middle of the day, and drinking alcohol in moderation.

Create a Bedtime Ritual

Reading, meditating, or taking a relaxing bath are all examples of activities that might send the message to the brain that it is time to wind down and relax. This activity right before bed has the potential to turn into a calming habit that gets the mind and body ready for sleep.

Exercise Regularly but Not Too Late in the Day

However, the timing of your workouts is really important for optimal sleep health. It's possible that doing vigorous exercise too close to bedtime will keep you awake. Finding the perfect balance and making time for exercise are both important factors in getting a good night's sleep.

Manage Stress

Anxiety can be reduced by practicing stress management techniques such as deep breathing, keeping a journal, or talking about your feelings with a trusted friend or a trained professional.

Optimize the Sleep Environment

As was mentioned before, the quality of one's sleep can be

improved by creating an atmosphere that is cozy and peaceful. Think about things like the temperature, the lighting, and the amount of noise.

Be Mindful of Naps

Naps of any length can be invigorating, but those taken too late in the day or for too long could make it difficult to fall or stay asleep at night. If you feel the need to nap, make sure they are short and taken earlier in the day.

Seek Professional Help if Needed

Insomnia that continues for an extended period should probably be evaluated by a specialist. Sleep specialists can give individualized therapy and techniques if they are required.

Consider the Needs of Others

If you sleep with a spouse, it is important to take into consideration their sleeping habits and preferences. Both parties can benefit from honest communication and being willing to make concessions to have a peaceful night's sleep.

Adults must do more than just put their heads on the pillow to make progress toward improved sleep quality. It calls for an approach that is comprehensive and takes into account lifestyle, habits, and individual requirements. The practice of mindfulness in all aspects of life, from daily routines to eating, has been shown to greatly improve the quality of sleep, which in turn leads to improvements in physical health, mental clarity, and overall life satisfaction.

A path can be paved toward consistent and restorative sleep by first acknowledging the specific obstacles that adults encounter and then addressing those challenges using the individualized solutions presented here. These recommendations are not simply a sleeping pill regimen; rather, they outline a way of life that incorporates sleep as a crucial component of overall health and well-being.

Tips for Children

It is essential for the growth, development, and overall health of children to ensure that they get a proper amount of sleep each night. The following are some strategies that parents and other caregivers can use to help youngsters meet their sleep requirements. Here are some suggestions that might help.

Establish a Consistent Sleep Schedule

Children thrive when they have a set schedule. Even on the weekends, maintaining a regular bedtime and wake-up time helps set one's internal body clock. Because of this regularity, it is easier for them to go to sleep and wake up in the morning.

Create a Calming Bedtime Routine

A calming pre-sleep ritual can send a message to a child's brain that it is time to start winding down and get ready for sleep. This routine could consist of activities such as reading a tale, having a warm bath, or listening to gentle music.

Optimize the Sleep Environment

Better sleep can be promoted by creating an environment that is cozy, free from disturbances, and conducive to rest. Think about things like the temperature of the room, how soft the bedding is, and how dim the lighting is. Children who are terrified of the dark may benefit from using nightlights in their rooms.

Avoid Screen Time Before Bed

Children are impacted by the blue light that is emitted by screens in the same way that adults are. Melatonin is the hormone responsible for inducing sleep. Helping the body's natural production of melatonin by avoiding stimulating activities such as television, computers, and tablets one hour before bedtime.

Encourage Physical Activity

A child's ability to fall asleep and stay asleep at night can be improved by engaging in active play and exercise during the day.

However, you should try to avoid engaging in strenuous activity in the hours leading up to night because it may be too stimulating.

Be Mindful of Food and Drink

A child's sleep can be made more restful if they avoid eating large meals, snacking on sugary foods, and drinking caffeinated beverages close to bedtime.

Provide a Comfort Item if Needed

Reassurance and relief from the stress associated with bedtime can be provided to younger children by using a comfort object, such as a cherished stuffed animal or blanket.

Communicate About Sleep

Encourage children to talk about any worries or concerns they have about going to bed, and engage them in dialogues about the significance of getting enough sleep.

Limit Naps for Older Children

While younger children need their naps, older children may benefit from having fewer or no naps at all, which can make it easier for them to go to sleep at night.

Respond to Nighttime Waking Calmly

If a child wakes up in the middle of the night, reassuring them and being calm is the best way to get them back to sleep without causing them distress. The treatment of these awakenings requires consistency, which is the key.

Seek Professional Help if Needed

Consultation with a pediatric sleep specialist may be necessary if sleep difficulties persist. They can evaluate the circumstance and offer solutions that are adapted to the child's particular requirements.

To be able to support a child's sleep, one must first understand the specific needs of the child and then put into action measures that nurture a good sleep routine. The provision of direction and the reassurance that is required by children falls primarily on the shoulders of the parents and other adults who are responsible for their care.

The implementation of these suggestions into daily life not only assures that children will experience restorative sleep, but also provides the groundwork for healthy sleeping habits that can last a person's entire life. Families can build an approach to rest that promotes their children's growth, learning, and happiness if they make sleep a priority and are sensitive to their individual children's needs and habits.

Special Considerations for Children with Special Needs

Children with physical, developmental, or behavioral issues may have their own set of difficulties falling or staying asleep. Their sleep requirements may be different, and it may be more difficult to accommodate these varying requirements. The following is an examination of methods and suggestions for facilitating restful sleep in children who have unique needs.

Understanding the Specific Needs

The distinctive demands of each child are distinct, and it is of the utmost importance to comprehend these requirements. Sleep can be affected by a variety of factors, including but not limited to medical issues, developmental disorders, and sensory sensitivities. To understand these individual requirements, working together with healthcare providers, therapists, or special educators is a good idea. This can help lead to proper sleep practices.

Develop a Tailored Sleep Routine

Bedtime routines that are highly regulated and predictable may be beneficial for children with special needs. Although routine is crucial for all children, children with special needs especially benefit from having one. To get a youngster ready for bed, it is often helpful to use things like visual calendars, tactile clues, or specialized rituals.

Create a Sensory-Friendly Environment

Children who have issues with their sense of touch, sight, hearing, or vision may require special consideration when it comes to the textures, colors, sounds, and lighting of their sleeping environment. You may need to make use of customized lighting, white noise devices, calming hues, and soft bedding.

Consider Medication and Dietary Factors

Children dealing with specific medical disorders may be prescribed medicines that disrupt their sleep. There is also the possibility that dietary limitations or particular nutritional requirements play a part. It is essential, to gain an understanding of these aspects, to consult with healthcare specialists.

Utilize Adaptive Equipment if Necessary

Children with physical limitations may need specialized bedding or seating arrangements to sleep peacefully. Therapists who specialize in occupational or physical therapy can be of assistance in evaluating and carrying out the implementation of these standards.

Provide Clear Communication

Children who have difficulties communicating may benefit from the use of language that is straightforward and uncomplicated, as well as from the provision of visual cues or assistive technology when discussing sleep routines and expectations.

Focus on Emotional Support

Children who have special needs may experience increased anxiety or terror in the hours before going to bed. Caregivers need to provide emotional support, compassion, and empathy to their patients.

Monitor Sleep Patterns

Keeping a sleep diary to record your sleeping patterns, as well as any difficulties or shifts you experience, might provide insightful information. More precise interventions may result from sharing this information with healthcare providers.

Engage in Collaborative Care

Collaboration with a group of sleep experts, such as pediatricians, therapists, and teachers of students with special needs, enables a well-rounded strategy for meeting the requirements of the child's sleep.

Educate Siblings and Other Family Members

It is possible to foster a more unified attitude to sleep within the family by providing the other members with an explanation of the special considerations and by including them in the routines.

Consider Professional Sleep Consultation

If difficulties falling or staying asleep continue, it may be good to seek the assistance of a sleep specialist who has prior experience working with children who have special needs.

It is necessary to take a sophisticated and tailored strategy in order to meet the sleeping requirements of children who have special needs. Parents and other caregivers can create a sleeping environment that caters to the specific requirements of the kid if they work together with trained specialists, implement individualized tactics, and provide consistent emotional support.

This process, despite the possibility that it may demand additional effort and patience, makes a substantial contribution to the child's general growth as well as their health and well-being. Children who have a wide range of requirements may benefit from having specialized interventions and daily routines designed to establish a secure and reassuring sleep environment. This results in improved rest for the kid and a deeper bond between the child and caregiver.

3.
INTRODUCTION TO BREATHING EXERCISES

Breathing exercises are one sometimes disregarded component when it comes to enhancing sleep. But what do breathing exercises entail, and how might they improve your ability to sleep? Let's get started by learning about the advantages of breathing exercises, how to begin doing them, and some specific exercises you can attempt to enhance your sleep.

What Are Breathing Exercises?

Relaxation and improved sleep can both be fostered via the practice of various breathing techniques. Finding out exactly what these exercises are, how they function, and how to put them into practice can lead to considerable increases in the quality of sleep one gets.

The term "breathing exercises" refers to a collection of practices that include the deliberate control and modification of one's breath. The basic goals of these exercises are to help participants relax, lessen feelings of stress, improve their ability to focus, and boost their general sense of well-being. Breathing exercises can help prepare the mind and body for rest, which can allow for a more seamless transition into sleep. When applied to the context of sleeping, several activities can have this effect.

Connection to Mind-Body Practices

Breathing exercises are frequently mentioned in conjunction with other mind-body disciplines such as mindfulness meditation, yoga, and others. These links have their origin in the realization that a state of mind that is calm and centered can be achieved via the use of controlled and focused breathing. The ability to exercise control over one's breath results in improved regulation of one's emotions as well as increased physical relaxation.

Different Types of Breathing Exercises

There are many different breathing exercises, each of which has its own distinct approach and objective. The following are some examples of common exercises:

Deep Breathing

This method of breathing, which is also known as diaphragmatic breathing, is taking long, slow breaths via the nose, allowing the lungs to become completely full, and then expelling slowly. This procedure promotes a thorough exchange of oxygen and slows down the rate at which the heart beats.

4-7-8 Technique

This well-known breathing exercise entails taking a breath in for four seconds, then holding it for seven seconds, and then releasing it for eight seconds. It is well known for the relaxing effects that it has.

Box Breathing

In this method, you take a breath in, hold it, exhale, and then take another breath in while holding it for an equal number of counts, typically four. It is frequently used to help people concentrate better and feel less anxious.

Belly Breathing

This technique encourages slower, more relaxed breathing by directing attention during inhalation to the expansion of the belly rather than the chest.

Integrating Breathing Exercises into Sleep Routines

Breathing exercises can be a helpful aid for people who

have trouble falling or staying asleep, especially if they are incorporated into a nightly routine. These exercises can be performed while seated in a relaxed position or while lying in bed, and they often only take a few minutes to complete. Getting assistance in learning and applying these skills can be done through facilitated seminars, mobile applications, or by working with a trained professional.

There is more to breathing exercises than simply inhaling and exhaling deeply; rather, they offer an all-encompassing method for achieving mind and body well-being. The benefits to one's mental and physical health that can result from gaining an understanding of and incorporating these exercises into one's daily routine, particularly in relation to sleep, can be substantial.

The act of practicing controlled breathing creates a pathway toward relaxation, renewal, and improved quality of life by acting as a bridge between the conscious and unconscious minds. Breathing exercises provide solutions that are both easy to implement and highly successful for achieving a variety of wellness goals, including better sleep, decreased stress, and overall improved well-being.

Benefits of Breathing Exercises

Exercises that focus on the breath are renowned for their numerous advantages that cut across both the physical and mental realms. These exercises go beyond simple relaxation techniques; they have been shown by science to improve general health and well-being. These are the main advantages:

Stress Reduction

The parasympathetic nervous system is triggered by breathing exercises, causing the body to relax. People can lower stress chemicals like cortisol by actively managing their breathing, which promotes peace and tranquility. Exercises such as the 4-7-8 approach are frequently used to swiftly relieve acute stress.

Improvement in Sleep Quality

Breathing exercises can greatly improve the quality of sleep because they relax you. They calm racing thoughts and release tense muscles to get the body and mind ready for sleep. People who struggle with insomnia or irregular sleep patterns may find techniques like deep breathing to be especially helpful.

Enhanced Emotional Well-being

Breathing exercises can improve emotional resilience and awareness. By concentrating on the breath, people can gain a sense of stability, which improves their ability to control their emotions. This knowledge frequently results in a happier mood and less anxiety.

Support for Respiratory Health

The respiratory system may benefit therapeutically from conscious breath regulation. It can enhance general lung health, expand lung capacity, and increase oxygenation. The benefits of breathing exercises may be especially beneficial for people with respiratory diseases like asthma.

Cardiovascular Health Benefits

Breathing exercises can enhance heart health by reducing stress and increasing oxygenation. They can support heart rate variability, lower blood pressure, and improve circulation. These outcomes support long-term cardiovascular health.

Pain Management

Some people find that doing breathing exercises can help them manage their chronic pain. They might experience less pain if they use relaxation techniques and concentrate on their breathing. This method is frequently applied in conjunction with other pain relief techniques.

Enhanced Concentration and Focus

Exercises that include controlled breathing, like box breathing, have been shown to improve focus and mental clarity. People can improve their focus and cognitive function by using their breath to anchor their minds to the present.

Support for Digestive Health

Exercises that involve breathing might, surprisingly, improve digestion. The digestive system's function can be enhanced by the relaxation response, which can increase blood flow there. Better digestion and nutrition absorption may result from this.

Complementary to Other Therapies

Yoga, meditation, and other forms of therapy, as well as psychotherapy, can all use breathing exercises. They can add a layer of calmness and mindfulness to these techniques to increase their efficacy.

Breathing exercises have a wealth of advantages beyond simply soothing the mind. They have the ability to improve many facets of health, including digestive support, emotional balance, physical health, and mental well-being. These exercises are adaptable tools that are simple to implement into daily routines. They can be used to improve sleep or increase focus.

They represent easily available, non-pharmaceutical therapies that can greatly improve people of all ages' quality of life and wellness. Breathing exercises are effective allies in fostering health and harmony within oneself, whether they are used as part of a sleep routine, stress management technique, or a holistic approach to well-being.

Getting Started with Breathing Exercises

It is a gratifying experience that can have a lot of positive effects on your health to start adding breathing exercises into your everyday life. Here is a starting point guide:

Understanding the Purpose

Determine your goals for your breathing exercises. Is it stress relief, improved sleep, increased attention, or another benefit?

Knowing your objective can aid you in choosing the best tactics to use.

Find a Comfortable Space

Select an area that is peaceful and comfortable and where you won't be bothered. It might be a quiet nook in your house or simply a bench in the park. You should be able to concentrate entirely on your breath since the environment should be serene.

Adopt a Comfortable Position

If sitting or lying down is more comfortable for you, choose that position. Maintain a straight back and calm hands. If it helps you concentrate, close your eyes.

Start with Simple Techniques

Start with simple breathing exercises like belly breathing or deep breathing if you're new to them. Here is a straightforward process to use:

- Take a few deep breaths in through your nose, and feel your stomach getting bigger as you do so.
- Attempt to hold your breath for a few seconds.
- Slowly let the air out of your lungs through your lips as you allow your abdominal muscles to tighten.
- Continue carrying out these steps for a period of several minutes.

Focus on Quality, Not Quantity

It is preferable to take your time with one breathing exercise rather than rushing through several. Quality training will increase the benefits and improve the experience.

Use Technology If Needed

Breathing exercises are demonstrated in several applications and videos. These resources might be quite beneficial if you find it difficult to handle them on your own.

Consistency is Key

Breathing exercises need to be consistently practiced, just like any other skill. An important difference can be made with just a few minutes per day. Pick a time that works for your schedule, and keep to it.

Monitor Your Progress

Record your feelings both before and after each session so that you may compare them. It can be quite motivating to see changes in your attitude, stress levels, or sleep patterns.

Explore Different Techniques

Once you're at ease with the fundamentals, you might want to investigate additional practices like guided meditations, the 4-7-8 approach, or box breathing. These may provide various benefits and experiences.

Consult Professionals if Necessary

Consider speaking with a therapist, yoga instructor, or another qualified specialist in breathwork if you have specific health concerns or if you wish to go deeper into breathing exercises.

Breathing exercises don't require specialized gear or in-depth training to begin. You can easily adapt this technique to meet your requirements and interests. You will be well on your way to enjoying the myriad benefits that this age-old practice has to offer if you begin with straightforward approaches and progressively investigate more involved practices as you progress.

Breathing exercises are a flexible and powerful tool for achieving these goals, whether you're trying to get more rest, lessen stress, or just feel better overall. Take your time and be sure to enjoy the ride because remember that persistence, patience, and consistency are the keys to your future success.

Breathing Exercises to Improve Sleep

The main goals of breathing exercises for better sleep are to relax the body and mind to get ready for a restful sleep. These exercises can be very beneficial for people who from insomnia or who just want to get a better night's sleep. Here is a closer look at a few efficient methods:

Progressive Relaxation

This method calls for successively tensing and relaxing various muscle groups. It can aid in releasing physical tension when combined with deep breathing:

- Deeply inhale, then contract a certain muscle group, such as the hands or feet.
- Release the tension in that muscle group as you slowly exhale.
- Repeat the technique as you move through the body's various components.

The 4-7-8 Method

It's commonly known that this practice helps people unwind and sleep better:

- Take a four-count while inhaling through your nose.
- Hold your breath for seven counts.
- Count to eight while exhaling through your lips.
- 3–4 times should be added to this cycle.

Diaphragmatic Breathing (Belly Breathing)

This practice, which involves using the diaphragm, encourages relaxation by emphasizing long, calm breaths:

- With both hands, place one on the abdomen and the other on the chest.
- Slowly inhale through your nose while allowing your stomach to expand.
- Gently exhale through the lips, allowing the abdominal muscles to tighten.
- For several minutes, do this while maintaining a rhythmic, even breath.

Guided Meditation and Visualization

This method involves listening to guided audio that instructs you to picture serene scenes or practice particular breathing techniques:

- Look for a guided meditation that is intended for sleep.
- Follow the directions while allowing the sounds and sights to calm your mind.

Humming Bee Breath (Bhramari Pranayama)

The following yoga exercise can help to relax the mind:

- Put your fingers on your forehead and use your thumbs to cover your ears.
- Deeply inhale using your nose.
- Exhale while producing a buzzing noise akin to a bee.
- Several times, repeat this.

Box Breathing

This technique can aid in relaxing you and regulating your breathing:

- Inhale for four counts.
- Hold your breath for four counts.
- Count to four as you exhale.
- Take a four-count pause.
- Proceed through multiple iterations of the process.

Exercises that focus on the breath can be quite effective in improving the quality of one's sleep. By putting these strategies into practice, individuals can cultivate a relaxing evening routine that sends cues to the body that it is time to unwind and relax before going to sleep. Consistent practice can lead to notable improvements in sleep quality, regardless of whether you opt for one strategy or a combination of methods.

To get the most out of the benefits of these exercises, it is best to do them in a serene setting free from any distractions and follow the instructions exactly. Always keep in mind that the keys to success in any new routine are patience and perseverance. These exercises may, with continued practice, eventually become an indispensable component of a restful and invigorating night's sleep.

4.

BREATHING EXERCISES FOR FAMILIES

The whole family may enjoy and benefit from teaching youngsters breathing techniques. They not only get better respiratory health and less stress, but they also pick up useful techniques that encourage mindfulness and self-awareness. Breathing exercises with your children can be a wonderful way to spend time together, promote calm, and establish lifelong healthy habits.

Why Practice with Your Kids?

Let's look at the **importance** of breathing exercises in the context of the family, especially with kids. Engaging in breathing exercises can enhance overall health and strengthen familial bonds.

Bonding and Connection

Breathing exercises offer a shared experience that might help parents and kids become more close. Together, participating in these activities fosters a special bonding experience where both parties can advance and encourage one another. It enables families to spend time together in a meaningful way, strengthening their emotional bond.

Emotional Regulation

Understanding and controlling emotions in children can be difficult. They can acquire tools to help them calm down during episodes of anxiety, rage, or irritation by practicing breathing techniques. Parents can provide guidance and encouragement by modeling appropriate emotional coping mechanisms and by practicing these strategies together.

Stress Reduction

Stress impacts both adults and children in today's fast-paced environment. All family members can reduce stress using easy-to-use breathing exercises. It's a useful coping strategy that may be used in a variety of circumstances, from exam jitters to nighttime anxiousness.

Enhancing Focus and Concentration

Children, especially those still developing, may have trouble focusing and paying attention. Breathing exercises aid in the development of mindfulness, improving the child's capacity for sustained attention. Their success in school and other areas of their lives that call for continuous focus may benefit from this improved attention span.

Encouraging Healthy Habits

Early exposure to breathing exercises instills healthy habits in kids that can last a lifetime. Children are more likely to continue practicing mindfulness and relaxation techniques as adults if these activities are encouraged in childhood. This foundation might result in a lifetime appreciation for self-care, mindfulness, and well-being in general.

Adaptation and Customization

Parents can modify workouts to fit their child's unique requirements and preferences by practicing with their kids. Parents might come up with interesting and enjoyable modifications to keep their child's attention and enthusiasm. These unique additions can help the child appreciate and benefit from the exercise more.

Improving Sleep Patterns

Previous chapters have demonstrated that breathing exercises have a significant impact on improving the quality of sleep. Implementing these exercises will help families who are having trouble with bedtime rituals establish a relaxing ritual that will help parents and kids go to sleep more easily.

Building Empathy and Understanding

Parents gain an understanding of their child's emotions and thinking through joint practice. Parents can better respond to their child's needs thanks to this awareness, which also builds empathy. By teaching kids to pay attention to their feelings, it also fosters empathy for others.

Breathing exercises are a technique that families may do together and reap a variety of advantages. It's an investment in the family's mental and physical well-being, from forging closer bonds to imparting crucial life skills. Making it a regular part of daily life for the family may foster harmony in the home and each family member's well-being.

Not only are the exercises important in and of themselves, but this practice also fosters relationships and teaches important life skills. Families who go on this collaborative journey not only improve the health of each member but also deepen the ties that bind them.

Exercises You Can Do Together

Here are some simple breathing exercises that families may do together to enjoy the many benefits of practicing deep breathing. These activities encourage a sense of community and shared experience while being entertaining for both adults and kids.

Balloon Breaths

An enjoyable exercise where participants visualize inflating and deflating a balloon with each breath. Children may find the exercise more interesting as a result of these images. This is how you do it:

- Either on the floor or on chairs, take a seat comfortably next to your youngster.
- Encourage your child to follow suit by placing their hands on their stomach.
- Imagine your stomach as a balloon inflating with air when you take a deep breath.
- Breathe out slowly while picturing the balloon deflating.
- Repeat numerous times while enlisting your kid's cooperation.

Benefits

Boosts lung capacity, induces mental calmness, and forges a fun relationship between participants.

Animal Breaths

Children can simulate the breathing rhythms of several animals with this imaginative activity. It's a terrific technique to add enjoyment and relatability to breathing exercises. This is how you do it:

- Choose one animal—a snake, a rabbit, an elephant— together.
- Discuss and demonstrate the animal's breathing pattern.
- For instance, a snake may breathe slowly before hissing loudly when it exhales.
- Repeat a few times, trying with other animals each time.

Benefits

Activates the imagination, contributes to the healthy management of emotions, and strengthens bonds.

Counting Breaths

Participants in this straightforward yet powerful exercise count their breaths simultaneously. This method promotes mindfulness and concentration. This is how you do it:

- Relax as you are seated in the same position as your youngster.
- Take a deep breath for four counts, hold it for four counts, and then let it out for four counts.
- Repeat while encouraging your youngster to join you in the counting.

Benefits

Helps one become more focused, relaxes one more deeply, and teaches one to be more patient.

Partner Breathing

Parents and kids must breathe in unison during this activity to create a shared experience. This is how you do it:

- As you breathe, sit back-to-back with your child and feel each other's backs.
- Make an effort to time your breaths as you inhale and exhale.
- Practice for a while, paying attention to how your breathing patterns interact.

Benefits

Improves the emotional connection, helps to build trust, and stimulates empathy in the recipient.

Guided Relaxation

A soothing activity in which one family member leads the others on a tranquil, imaginative journey while utilizing setting-specific terminology. This is how you do it:

- One individual talks about a calm environment, like a beach or forest.
- Others listen while picturing the situation and paying attention to their breathing.

- Change duties so that each family member can guide in turn.

Benefits

Boosts creativity, encourages relaxation, and provides opportunities for one-of-a-kind shared experiences.

These activities provide families with a fun and beneficial way to bond, unwind, and develop as a unit. These joint activities allow parents and kids to forge closer bonds, teach important coping mechanisms, and forge enduring memories. Each exercise has a special offering that meets various interests and requirements. By incorporating these activities into daily life, families can feel more connected and at ease, which contributes to a happier, more loving home.

Tips for Success

It's crucial to look at various methods that may be effective while engaging in breathing exercises with your family. These recommendations are intended to improve the encounter and make it more pleasurable, efficient, and long-lasting for everyone involved.

Start Slow

It's crucial to start slowly and build up the practice over time, especially if you or your kids are new to breathing exercises.

Advice

Start with briefer sessions and easy exercises. As everyone feels more at ease, gradually up the duration and complexity.

Make it a Routine

Breathing exercises might be significantly more helpful when they are performed consistently.

Advice

Set up a certain time every day, such as right before bed or right after school, to practice. As much as you can, follow the schedule to create a habit.

Use Props and Visuals

Children will find exercises more fascinating and will comprehend subjects more clearly with the aid of props and images.

Advice

To illustrate the exercises, use balloons, plush animals, or photos. Give kids the option to select their props to increase excitement and a sense of involvement.

Be Patient and Supportive

A calm and nurturing atmosphere can be produced with patience and support.

Advice

As kids learn and practice, give them encouragement and praise. Be forgiving of errors or problems and offer gentle direction.

Modify as Needed

Flexibility can make the experience better because each family member may have different wants or preferences.

Advice

Exercises can be modified to fit various age groups, skill levels, or interests. Encourage criticism and show flexibility in adapting to personal preferences.

Lead by Example

Kids typically pick up knowledge by watching adults. Setting a good example can be a very effective teaching strategy.

Advice

Self-exercise is encouraged, as is a positive attitude about the activities. Talk to your kids about your experiences and what you like most about the practice.

Focus on Enjoyment

Adding enjoyment and fun to the exercise will probably boost dedication and enthusiasm.

Advice

Include activities, tales, or themes that speak to your kids. Encourage creativity and humor while doing the activities.

Communicate Openly

Collaboration and understanding are promoted by open communication.

Advice

With your family, talk about your hopes, feelings, and ideas for the exercises. Encourage kids to voice their thoughts and consider them when making decisions.

Monitor Progress

Monitoring your development can inspire you and give you insightful information.

Advice

Take note of any modifications in your sleep, emotions, or behavior. Celebrate advancements and consider what benefits your family the most.

These pointers serve as a road map for effectively adopting breathing exercises in a family setting. Families can develop a meaningful and rewarding practice by taking into account individual requirements, keeping consistency, and putting the enjoyment of the activity first. Exploring breathing techniques together can strengthen bonds, improve health, and promote a happy and peaceful home life. The process of breathing together may be a rewarding adventure full of development, kinship, and love.

Tracking Progress Together

Families need to practice breathing exercises together as well as grow and develop as a unit. Together, tracking progress fosters a sense of accomplishment and keeps people motivated. We'll go over some strategies and advantages of monitoring your family's progress using breathing exercises below.

Why Monitor Progress?

Every practice, including breathing exercises, should include a way to monitor progress. In order to:

Measure Improvement

Recognize your progress and the changes that have occurred.

Maintain Motivation

Observe triumphs and look for places for improvement.

Customize Practice

Adapt the exercises to what your family finds to be most effective.

Foster Connection

Make learning and success an experience that everyone can share.

Methods for Tracking Progress

Establish a Progress Journal

Journaling about your family's experience with breathing exercises can be interesting and instructive.

How to Implement

- Set aside a journal or electronic document for progress logging.
- Encourage all members of the family to share their experiences through writing or art.
- Include information such as the time, exercises done, emotions, and observations.

Use a Visual Chart

For younger children, a visual chart can be an interesting method to track growth.

How to Implement

- Make a chart to depict various milestones using stickers, colors, or symbols.

- To make the chart dynamic, invite kids to contribute to its update.

Set Goals and Milestones

Setting definite, attainable goals provides your practice direction.

How to Implement

- Specify clear goals, such as mastering a particular workout or getting better sleep.
- When objectives are achieved, reminisce about the factors that made them possible.

Regular Family Discussions

Check-ins at regular intervals foster an open discourse regarding developments, difficulties, and emotions.

How to Implement

- Set up regular family gatherings to talk about what's working and what needs to be changed.
- Take into account one another's viewpoints and act as a group.

Utilize Apps or Tools

Technology can offer a methodical way to monitor progress.

How to Implement

- Investigate applications with tracking capabilities for breathing exercises or mindfulness.
- Together, review your progress and go over any themes you've noticed.

Considerations and Tips

Individualize Tracking

Recognize that it's okay if each family member develops at a different rate.

Encourage Honesty

Establish a secure environment where people can open up about their genuine experiences.

Celebrate Together

Celebrate successes as a family to promote optimism.

Stay Flexible

Be prepared to modify your strategies or objectives as you discover what works best for your family.

An effective technique to increase the family's involvement in breathing exercises is to track progress together. It encourages a sense of cohesion and direction and aids in adjusting the practice to the particular dynamics of your family. You can make the experience rich and gratifying for everyone involved by accepting this shared adventure and appreciating each step along the way. It transforms practicing breathing exercises into a shared family journey full of learning, development, and connection from a straightforward activity.

5.
INTRODUCTION TO MEDITATION

Since ancient times, people have utilized meditation as a potent tool to create mental clarity, lower stress, enhance sleep, and enhance general well-being. Finding calm and quiet in today's hectic environment can be difficult, which is why meditation should be a regular part of any self-care regimen.

What Is Meditation?

Let's look into meditation, a tradition that spans generations and cultural boundaries. This chapter will lay the groundwork for understanding the various aspects of meditation and its applicability in the modern world.

Meditation is a form of mental exercise that entails concentration, relaxation, and awareness of one's surroundings. It is the practice of focusing one's attention on a single object, thought, or action to improve one's attention and awareness, as well as achieve a condition that is mentally clear as well as emotionally tranquil and stable. Meditation aims to train one's attention in a more meaningful way, as opposed to the random thoughts that normally fill one's mind.

Historical Background

The practice of meditation has been around for a considerable number of centuries. It has its origins in several different religious and philosophical schools, including Buddhism, Hinduism, and Taoism. The concept was adopted and developed further by each culture, which resulted in a large number of distinct approaches and philosophies.

Types of Meditation

Numerous schools of thought and cultural canons have contributed to the development of a diverse range of meditative techniques. The following are examples of kinds that are quite common:

Mindfulness Meditation

Awareness of the present moment is emphasized, with a particular emphasis placed on paying attention to one's thoughts and feelings in a nonjudgmental manner.

Transcendental Meditation

Involves reciting a certain mantra to induce a state of profound mental relaxation in oneself.

Loving-Kindness Meditation

Fosters kindness and affection not only for oneself but also for other people.

Guided Meditation

The participant is led through a visualized experience either in person by a trained practitioner or remotely via an audio recording.

Movement-Based Meditation

Meditation can be achieved through the use of practices like Yoga and Tai Chi, which include adopting specific physical postures and focusing on one's breathing.

Purposes and Goals

People meditate for a variety of reasons, including the following:

Personal Growth

Increasing one's self-awareness while also improving one's emotional health and connectedness to the spiritual world.

Health Benefits

Reducing stress, anxiety, and sadness while also increasing heart health and quality of sleep are the goals of this therapy.

Enhanced Concentration

Enhancing one's ability to concentrate, remember information, and think clearly.

Connection to Others

Increasing caring, empathy, and comprehension of other people's perspectives and experiences.

Common Misconceptions

There are several myths surrounding the practice of meditation, such as the idea that one needs to entirely clear their mind or that one must sit in a certain way. The truth is that there is no "one size fits all" method of practicing meditation because it is highly malleable.

How to Get Started

Beginning a practice of meditation doesn't call for any specialized gear or substantial prior experience:

Find a Place to Be Alone

Reduce the number of things that can pull your focus away.

Pick an Approach to Do It

Choose an approach that speaks to you on some level.

Determine a Time

When it comes to building habits, consistency is key.

Have Patience!

It is not unusual to experience difficulties in the beginning. The key to success is perseverance.

Meditation is a multidimensional activity that has significant effects on one's mental health as well as emotional and physical well-being. Anyone willing to put in the necessary effort and put in the necessary amount of time can develop this skill. Individuals can engage on a personal path towards greater clarity, calm, and personal fulfillment by first gaining an awareness of what meditation actually is and then becoming familiar with the many forms and functions it can serve.

This short intro is a first step into the practice of meditation, which can lead to significant personal growth and a more meaningful engagement with the world.

How to Get Started with Meditation

It's beneficial to establish your goals before starting your meditation journey. Understanding your purpose can help you make decisions about the approaches and strategies that will help you achieve your objectives, whether they are stress reduction, improved focus, personal development, or spiritual exploration.

Selecting the Right Technique

There are many different kinds of meditation, as previously mentioned. Some people might choose present-centered mindfulness, while others may find resonance in mantra-based practices like Transcendental Meditation. Discovering many approaches and trying out a few will help you choose the one that feels most natural to you.

Finding Guidance

Self-directed meditation is an option, however, guided sessions are often more beneficial for beginners. These are available as books, online videos, or mobile applications. Numerous towns have live lessons taught by qualified professors, which can offer individualized advice.

Setting Up Your Space

It's essential to choose a peaceful, comfortable location where you won't be bothered when meditating if you want to stay focused. It doesn't have to be a dedicated space; even a calm nook with a cozy chair or cushion will do. Some individuals choose the addition of calming components like subdued lighting or relaxing background music.

Determining the Duration

The technique can be made more bearable by beginning with brief sessions (5-10 minutes) and progressively extending the length as you grow more comfortable. There is no set formula for the "right" duration; instead, it should correspond to how long it feels right to you.

Developing a Routine

In meditation, consistency is important. More significant advantages can result from choosing a set time of day and making meditation a regular habit. While some people find morning meditation to be the best time, others might prefer a lunchtime or evening session.

Practicing Mindfully

The mind frequently wanders while one is meditating. When this occurs, it's crucial to gently and without condemnation return your focus to it. It involves mental training, thus patience is needed.

Tracking Progress

Keeping a meditation notebook is beneficial for some people. Recording your thoughts, feelings, and experiences can provide you with a valuable perspective on your development and reveal areas in which you might wish to modify your practice.

Seeking Community

A local or online meditation group can provide support, inspiration, and the opportunity to exchange experiences. Engaging with individuals who are traveling a similar path can increase motivation and offer fresh perspectives.

It doesn't have to be difficult or daunting to begin meditating. You can start a satisfying and transforming journey by being aware of your objective, choosing the appropriate method, creating a supportive environment, and establishing regular habits.

Even though difficulties could arise, persistence, patience, and perhaps asking for advice from seasoned practitioners can all help to develop a fruitful meditation practice. Everyone has access to the path of meditation, which offers substantial advantages that can spread to other areas of life and improve general well-being.

Meditation Techniques for Better Sleep

Let's explore some specific meditation methods that can be used to enhance the quality of your sleep. These techniques aim to relax the body, quiet the mind, and promote restful sleep because they recognize the importance of sleep for general health.

Guided Sleep Meditation

Following a recorded meditation conducted by a teacher is part of guided sleep meditation. The advice frequently consists of calming exercises for the body and mind, such as visualization, positive affirmations, and relaxation techniques. This type of meditation can be available on several platforms, including applications and sleep-related YouTube channels.

Progressive Muscle Relaxation

Different muscle groups are tensed and then gradually released using this technique. The body can relax and the mind can be distracted from anxious thoughts by focusing on the relaxation. It is possible to thoroughly relax the body by starting at the toes and working your way up, which makes it easier to fall asleep.

Mindfulness Meditation

Focusing on the present moment is encouraged by mindfulness meditation. When using this technique to fall asleep, one may focus on their breathing, the feel of their bed, or the sounds in the room. The mind's chatter can be reduced and a tranquil state that is favorable to sleeping can be achieved by gently drawing attention back anytime it wanders.

Deep Breathing Techniques

The body's relaxation response can be triggered by deep breathing techniques like the 4-7-8 technique (inhale for 4 seconds, hold for 7, exhale for 8). The body can enter a tranquil state and get ready for sound sleep by concentrating on the breath and maintaining this pattern.

Yoga Nidra (Yogic Sleep)

Yoga Nidra is a type of conscious relaxation that is frequently used to improve sleep. Participants are brought to a condition between wakefulness and sleep by guided imagery and body scanning, which can make it easier to fall asleep. The process might be aided by certain recordings or classes that focus on Yoga Nidra for sleep.

Visualization Techniques

The mind can be diverted from tension or anxiety by picturing a serene setting, like a tranquil beach or forest. The more vivid the visual, the better the mind can relate to the soothing scene and ease into sleep.

Mantra Meditation

A relaxing word or phrase repeated out loud or in silence might help you focus during meditation and block out distracting ideas. You can make up your mantra or choose a classic one that has to do with relaxation or sleep.

Incorporating Sleep-Inducing Sounds

Some people discover that combining relaxing sounds, such as white noise, quiet music, or natural sounds, helps them achieve a meditative state that is beneficial to sleep. There are specialized recordings made with aural stimulation to enhance sleep meditation.

These numerous methods provide a wide range of meditation

strategies for bettering sleep. A practice that is customized to each client's needs and preferences can be developed by experimenting with various approaches and discovering what works. These methods used regularly, along with a comfortable sleeping environment and good sleep hygiene, can significantly improve sleep quality. These meditation techniques provide a complete route to sound sleep because they acknowledge the link between the mind and body.

Meditation Techniques You Can Do with Your Kids

Children can learn mindfulness and relaxation skills by being introduced to meditation techniques. The following methods promote a setting that promotes both relaxation and connection while being kid-friendly.

Animal Breathing Meditation

You can employ several breathing exercises with animal themes to make the meditation enjoyable for kids since they often have a strong connection to animals. For instance, you could exhort them to "roar like a lion" or "breathe like a snake" by exhaling deeply.

Story Meditation

It might be entertaining and comforting to write a calming story with visual components that kids can follow along with. A vivid and tranquil mental image can be created by leading them on a peaceful stroll through a garden, a forest, or along the beach.

Mindful Coloring or Drawing

Children can express themselves creatively while focused on the present moment by meditating while sketching or coloring. Give them some crayons and paper, and let them express themselves through drawing as they meditate or listen to relaxing music.

Bubble Breathing Exercise

Children can be encouraged to act like they are blowing bubbles. Tell them to inhale deeply and exhale slowly, as if they were blowing actual bubbles. Children find breathing exercises to be more interesting thanks to this creative approach.

The Gratitude Meditation

It can be a lovely practice to teach kids to be grateful. You can help them focus on feeling grateful by asking them to consider something for which they are grateful. This might be a daily bedtime habit.

Guided Imagery with Stuffed Animals

It can be more relaxing to include a child's favorite stuffed animal in a meditation. They can imagine the plush animal rising and falling with each breath while holding it and breathing in time with it.

The Sound Game

Close your eyes and listen to the sounds around you with your child, whether they are the distant sound of traffic or the rustle of the leaves. You can then talk about what you heard. It's an easy method to exercise being in the now.

Body Scanning with a Toy

Touch various regions of the child's body with a small toy (such as a plush feather or a toy car). Tell the child to concentrate on how each component feels as you touch it. This introduces body scanning in a haptic manner.

Flower and Candle Breathing

Tell your youngster to inhale while pretending their hand is a flower, smelling the fictitious flower, and to exhale while pretending their hand is a candle, blowing the candle. To help children learn to breathe deeply, say this aloud multiple times.

Partner Yoga and Meditation

Simple yoga poses and meditation can be practiced simultaneously for fun and to strengthen relationships. There are yoga poses that include meditation that are appropriate for kids.

These creative and entertaining methods for teaching meditation to kids can promote emotional awareness, calmness, and attention. Parents may provide their kids with useful strategies for managing stress and cultivating mindfulness by making the practices engaging and relatable for them.

Additionally, using these methods as a family strengthens the bond between parents and children and makes meditation a fun pastime for everyone. By investing in these techniques, you're fostering life skills that can help children in a variety of areas of their lives in addition to improving their sleep.

6.
ENHANCING SLEEP THROUGH MEDITATION

Our general health and happiness depend heavily on how well we sleep. Sleep disorders including insomnia, sleep apnea, and restless leg syndrome are unfortunately very common. Even if we don't have a sleep problem that has been officially diagnosed, we may still have trouble going to sleep, staying asleep, or receiving quality sleep. This is where meditation enters the picture; it has been demonstrated to enhance sleep quality and can be a potent technique in resolving sleep disorders.

How Meditation Improves Sleep

Focusing the mind, controlling breathing, and promoting a deep state of relaxation are all aspects of the meditation practice. It has proven to be a successful strategy for improving sleep quality over time. Let's look into how meditation accomplishes this, which makes it an indispensable tool for people who are trying to improve their quality of sleep:

Calming the Mind

Meditation is effective because it slows down the racing thoughts that frequently keep us up at night. Meditation aids in lowering worry and tension, two main causes of sleep disturbances, by teaching the mind to concentrate on the here and now. Through mindfulness exercises, one can learn to be more conscious of the thoughts and feelings that are present at any given time, making it easier to fall asleep peacefully.

Reducing Stress Hormones

According to studies, meditation can reduce cortisol and other stress hormones in the body. Reduced levels of these hormones cause the body's natural relaxation response to be activated, which helps to promote a calm state that is favorable to sleep. People who suffer from insomnia or other sleep issues linked to stress may find this to be of great benefit.

Enhancing Relaxation

Techniques for meditation frequently emphasize slow, rhythmic breathing and relaxed muscles. These techniques help the body into the ideal state of relaxation for sleep. One can more easily drift off to a comfortable sleep by deliberately relaxing various body regions.

Regulating the Sleep-Wake Cycle

It has been discovered that some types of meditation are beneficial for the circadian rhythm, which controls our sleep-wake cycle. One can encourage a sound sleep pattern and train the body to know when to wind down by meditating at the same time each day, preferably before bed.

Improving Sleep Quality

Not only can meditation aid in sleep onset, but it also improves sleep quality in general. People who regularly meditate frequently report sleeping longer and more deeply and waking up feeling more rested and energized.

Addressing Specific Sleep Disorders

To treat particular sleep disorders like nightmares or sleep apnea, meditation can be specifically adapted. People have used methods like guided imagery or mindfulness-based therapy to solve these specific difficulties, providing a healthy and non-invasive method of enhancing sleep.

Fostering a Bedtime Ritual

The mind and body can be told to get ready for sleep by including meditation in a nightly regimen. This custom establishes a routine that supports the body's predisposition to sleep at night.

Promoting Emotional Well-Being

Sleep quality is greatly influenced by the emotional balance that meditation encourages. Meditation aids in establishing a psychological setting conducive to more naturally occurring sleep by resolving underlying emotional problems.

Because it affects both the body and the mind, meditation is a comprehensive method for enhancing sleep quality. Meditation is a flexible and affordable method that anyone trying to improve their sleep may use to calm their mind, lower stress hormones, promote relaxation, and regulate sleep patterns.

It adds value to a sleep improvement plan and promotes a healthier, more balanced way of living due to its adaptability to individual demands. The effect of meditation on sleep, whether in adults or children, is proof of the effectiveness of mind-body techniques in enhancing general well-being.

Implementing Meditation into Your Routine

By including meditation in your daily routine, you can significantly improve your mental and physical health by sharpening your attention, lowering your stress levels, and promoting sounder sleep. You can easily incorporate meditation techniques into your daily life by following these steps:

Start Small

Start with brief meditation sessions if you are new to it. Every day for just 5 to 10 minutes can make an impact. As you become more accustomed to the exercise, gradually lengthen the time.

Find the Right Time and Place

Pick a time when you're least likely to be interrupted and when it works best for you. To start their day off well, many people choose to meditate in the morning, but you can do it whenever you like. Additionally, look for a calm, cozy area where you may relax.

Use Guided Meditations

Videos or applications that offer guided meditation can be a great resource, especially for beginners. You can maintain focus and give your practice structure by using a guide.

Create a Meditation Space

Your experience may be improved by having a special place set out for meditation. It doesn't have to be extravagant; just a calm area with a cozy chair or cushion would do. You can use relaxing components like plants or subdued lighting.

Be Consistent

To establish a habit, try to meditate at the same time each day. To reap the benefits of meditation over the long run, consistency is essential.

Involve Your Family

As was already said, families can participate in meditation. Meditating alongside your kids or partner can strengthen your relationship and promote a shared practice.

Experiment with Different Techniques

Try a few different meditation methods to find the one that appeals to you the most because not all of them will. The variety may keep your practice interesting, whether it's body scanning, mindfulness, or breathing exercises.

Combine Meditation with Other Activities

You can include meditation in routine tasks like eating, walking, and even taking a shower. Walking or eating mindfully can be a type of meditation in and of itself.

Keep a Meditation Journal

Following up with your thoughts and feelings after each session might help you keep track of your progress and gain insights into your mental health and development. Additionally, it can aid in further individualizing your practice.

Be Patient and Kind to Yourself

During meditation, if your mind wanders, don't be too hard on yourself. It is typical, especially when you first begin. Bring your focus back slowly and go on.

Seek Support if Needed

Consider attending a local meditation group or getting advice from a meditation instructor if you're having trouble meditating on your own.

It doesn't take a lot of effort or time to include meditation in your daily practice. You may develop a practice that fits into your daily life by beginning small and building up gradually. You may make meditation a fun and useful part of your life by involving family members, trying out various approaches, and discovering what works best for you.

It's a holistic approach to well-being that can have a good influence on a variety of elements of life, from relationships to personal development. It's not only about improving sleep. With time and effort, meditation can become a beneficial component of your daily routine that promotes both short-term well-being and long-term calm.

Guiding Children Through Meditation

For both the child and the parent or guardian, leading a child in meditation can be a rewarding experience. It can be a technique to aid youngsters in managing stress and fostering inner calm, emotional regulation, and focus.

Understand Their Needs and Interests

Depending on their age and personality, children's demands and interests might differ dramatically. Make the meditation activities specific to their individual needs. Talk to them about it to learn what they might find intriguing or comforting.

Start with Short Sessions

Children might find it difficult to sit quietly for prolonged periods of time, unlike adults. Start with little sessions, perhaps 2 to 5 minutes, and then progressively lengthen them as they feel more at ease.

Create a Calming Environment

Create a serene, silent area for meditation. Children may find the space more welcoming if there are plush pillows, low lighting, or relaxing background music.

Use Simple Techniques

Start with easy-to-follow meditation methods that are basic and enjoyable for kids. They may find engaging techniques like deep breathing or concentrating on an object.

Incorporate Imagery and Storytelling

Imaginative scenarios and stories frequently strike a chord with kids. Make a guided meditation that transports them to a serene location, like flying in the sky or meandering through a forest.

Be Patient and Positive

Children frequently become restless or preoccupied. Keep your mood upbeat and patient, and if they stray, gently bring them back.

Include Movement

There are many different techniques for meditation. Incorporating thoughtful exercises like stretches or yoga poses might be useful for more active kids.

Emphasize Sensory Experience

Children frequently focus heavily on their senses. Exercises that emphasize noises, sensations, or even tastes are acceptable. You could instruct them to experience the ring of a bell or the feel of soft cloth, for instance.

Provide Reassurance and Guidance

During meditation, kids may experience queries or emotions. Be there to reassure and direct them, assisting them in comprehending what they are going through.

Make It a Regular Practice

Children will gain more from frequent practice, just like adults do. Include meditation in your routine, possibly right before bed or right after school.

Celebrate Progress

Positive reinforcement is used to recognize and reward accomplishments. Encouragement from others or modest rewards can spur them to keep up the routine.

Include Them in Your Practice

If you practice meditation, bring them along when it makes sense. When they witness you meditating, your children may be inspired.

It takes imagination, tolerance, and an awareness of each child's particular needs and interests to guide them through meditation. You are assisting children in developing a talent that can be useful to them throughout their lives by making the process interesting, straightforward, and pleasurable.

Even though it could take some time for them to get fully involved in meditation, the effort you put forth to introduce children to this practice can create the groundwork for a habit of mindfulness and self-awareness that will last them their entire lives. Keep in mind that the objective is to foster a nice and relaxing experience that helps their emotional and mental well-being rather than perfection.

Measuring Improvements in Sleep

Measuring sleep improvement is a crucial component of assessing the efficacy of practices like meditation, breathing exercises, or other sleep-related activities. Finding out what is working and what needs more modification is helpful.

Keep a Sleep Journal

A sleep diary can be an effective tool for monitoring changes in sleep habits. Make notes about your bedtime, wake-up time, the total amount of sleep you get, the quality of your sleep, and any dreams or disturbances. Insights into the elements impacting sleep can also be gained by writing down emotions and thoughts before sleeping.

Use Technology

A thorough examination of sleep cycles, restfulness, and disruptions can be obtained using a variety of sleep-tracking gadgets and apps. These solutions frequently make use of sensors and algorithms to provide a more accurate measurement of sleep improvement and quality.

Observe Changes in Daytime Functioning

Better sleep frequently results in more effective daytime performance. Observe any changes in your mood, focus, energy level, and general health. Parents and other adults who are caring for children may notice behavioral improvements, such as improved academic focus or a happier mood.

Monitor Physical Health Indicators

Physical wellness is intimately correlated with sleep. Monitoring parameters like blood pressure, body mass index, or immune system activity can give indirect indications of sleep quality improvements.

Assess Children's Sleep Through Communication

Engaging children in dialogue about their feelings and dreams can reveal insights because children may not be able to express their sleep experiences as well as adults do. Younger children may convey their sleep experience through games or drawings, so pay attention to these covert cues.

Look for a Reduction in Sleep Problems

If specific sleep disorders were first recognized, monitoring their disappearance or diminution is a definite indicator of improvement. This may involve conditions including sleep apnea in youngsters, sleeplessness, night terrors, or frequent awakening in adults.

Consider Professional Assessment if Needed

Professional sleep studies performed by healthcare professionals can give a thorough review of sleep issues that persist or if a more in-depth investigation is requested.

Focus on Consistency

Consistency is more important for improving sleep than one or two exceptional nights. Instead of looking for sporadic fantastic nights, focus on patterns of consistent high-quality sleep.

Reflect on the Impact of Implemented Techniques

Take into account how practices like meditation or breathing exercises are affecting the quality of your sleep. Depending on how each person responds to these techniques, adjustments can be made.

Involve Children in the Process

Use engaging methods to involve kids when assessing sleep improvement. Make a sleep log they can complete or incorporate into a game. This may increase their interest in the tracking procedure.

A holistic strategy that takes into account many physical, emotional, and behavioral components is needed to measure improvements in sleep. It is possible to evaluate the efficacy of programs targeted at improving sleep by combining subjective observations, technology instruments, professional assessment, and incorporating kids in a kid-friendly way.

It's a method that encourages not only better sleep but also a deeper awareness of individual sleep needs and responses, supporting ongoing efforts to establish a regular sleep schedule that is both healthy and restorative.

7.
STRATEGIES FOR SPECIAL NEEDS CHILDREN

Sleep is critical for the development of all children, even those with unique requirements. On the other hand, children who have special needs frequently deal with one-of-a-kind obstacles, which might make it difficult for them to acquire the necessary amount of peaceful sleep.

Understanding Specific Needs (e.g., ADHD)

Children with particular requirements, such as Attention Deficit Hyperactivity Disorder (ADHD), Autism Spectrum Disorder (ASD), sensory processing abnormalities, and other neurological or developmental variations, must get extra consideration while treating their sleep needs. These particular needs can make it difficult to get a good night's sleep, but they can be overcome with awareness and specially designed techniques. The following information on how particular needs, such as ADHD, may affect sleep and how to support these kids

ADHD and Sleep Challenges

Impulsivity, hyperactivity, and trouble paying attention are symptoms of Attention Deficit Hyperactivity Disorder (ADHD). Children with ADHD frequently experience difficulties sleeping. Some of the difficulties people might have sleeping include:

Difficulty Falling Asleep

A youngster with ADHD may have trouble winding down for bed since they are so active and restless.

Restless Sleep

Children with ADHD may wake up more frequently during the night and may find it more difficult to fall back asleep.

Impact on Behavior and Learning

Lack of sleep can make ADHD symptoms worse, making academic and behavioral issues during the day more severe.

Understanding Other Specific Needs

There may be particular sleep difficulties for kids with other special needs, such as Autism Spectrum Disorder or sensory processing issues. These could result from inflexible habits, communication issues, or sensory sensitivities. In order to develop a successful sleep strategy, it is essential to comprehend the special difficulties connected to each need.

Tailored Strategies for Specific Needs

A tailored strategy is necessary to assist kids with special needs in getting quality sleep. The following tactics could be useful:

Establishing a Routine

By establishing a regular bedtime routine, you can help your child understand when it's time to relax and get ready for bed.

Providing Sensory Supports

A tranquil sleep environment can be created for kids with sensory sensitivity by integrating sensory-friendly items like weighted blankets or relaxing music.

Behavioral Interventions

Teaching behaviors connected to sleep can be accomplished with the help of strategies like positive reinforcement or the use of visual timetables.

Professional Guidance

Insight into customized tactics and actions can be gained by speaking with specialists who are aware of the particular need.

Collaboration with Professionals and Caregivers

Collaboration between parents, educators, therapists, and other professionals who are aware of the child's specific requirements is essential for providing effective care for children with special needs. Collaboration and information exchange can result in a well-thought-out strategy that encourages healthier sleep.

Using Medication Thoughtfully

To address sleep issues, medication may be recommended in some circumstances. However, it's crucial to proceed cautiously, speaking with medical professionals to make sure the drug is suitable, and keeping an eye out for any potential adverse effects.

Children with special needs, such as ADHD, face particular difficulties getting a good night's sleep, but these difficulties can be overcome with compassion, teamwork, and specialized approaches. Working with a supportive team and taking into account each child's unique needs and features can result in a successful sleep plan that improves general well-being.

An environment that is more supportive of sound sleep and a happier, healthier child can be achieved by highlighting the value of a holistic approach that includes environmental changes, behavioral techniques, and expert coaching.

Tailored Strategies for Better Sleep

Children with special needs, such as ADHD, Autism Spectrum Disorder, sensory processing issues, or other particular conditions, have different sleep needs than regular kids. It is crucial to develop solutions that are customized for each child as a result. An examination of ways to modify sleep techniques is provided below:

Assessing Individual Needs

Understanding the child's unique requirements, preferences, and obstacles is crucial first and foremost. This may entail figuring out the child's sensory sensitivities, comprehending his or her daily schedule, identifying any illnesses, and figuring out any particular worries or anxieties the child may have regarding sleep.

Creating a Supportive Sleep Environment

The atmosphere in the bedroom is quite important for fostering restful sleep. Customized tactics could include:

Sensory Considerations

The bedroom can be made to feel cozier by utilizing soothing hues, plush materials, and tranquil sounds.

Accessibility

The space can be made more pleasant by arranging the bedroom to accommodate the child's physical requirements or limits.

Personal Preferences

The child's favorite themes or items might be incorporated to create a cozy and comfortable atmosphere in the room.

Establishing Consistent Bedtime Routines

For many children with exceptional needs, routine is essential. Customized bedtime rituals could consist of:

Visual Schedules

Children can better grasp the nighttime routine by being shown photos of it.

Incorporating Favorite Activities

A favorite story or relaxation technique can add to the fun of bedtime.

Collaborating with Professionals

Therapists, educators, and healthcare professionals who are knowledgeable about the child's particular requirements can offer priceless insights into customized approaches. The techniques will be in line with the child's overall care plan if these professionals are involved in the collaboration.

Using Technology and Tools

Technology or assistive equipment may be useful in some situations. This may consist of:

Adaptive Bedding

Mattresses or pillows are specifically made to meet physical needs.

Monitoring Devices

tools to monitor sleep habits and spot potential issues.

Incorporating Behavioral Strategies

A child's unique issues can be taken into account when designing behavioral interventions:

Positive Reinforcement

Consistency can be encouraged by rewarding good sleeping patterns.

Gradual Changes

A gradual change in bedtime or habit might make transitions easier.

Educating and Involving the Family

Family members are essential in putting customized sleep techniques into practice. By giving them the required knowledge, assistance, and resources, you can make sure that the techniques are applied consistently.

Ongoing Evaluation and Adjustment

Continuous evaluation and modification of sleep techniques are essential since children's demands alter as they mature and develop. The techniques will remain efficient and applicable as long as there is regular communication with experts, tracking of progress, and a willingness to make the required adjustments.

Customizing sleep strategies for children with exceptional needs necessitates a thorough comprehension of their particular needs, teamwork with experts, and a flexible, tailored approach. These techniques can improve sleep quality, boost overall development, and promote a more peaceful family life by concentrating on the child's particular requirements and collaborating closely with a helpful team.

These customized approaches recognize the child's individuality and work to offer the most supportive and efficient sleep solutions, whether through alterations to the environment, behavioral techniques, or collaboration with specialists.

Supporting Parents and Caregivers

Taking care of a child with special needs frequently presents particular difficulties, particularly when it comes to sleep. To cross this difficult terrain, parents and caregivers require specialized equipment, strategies, and emotional support. A breakdown of how to assist them is provided below:

Providing Education and Training

Understanding is a useful tool. The first step toward enabling parents and caregivers to promote better sleep can be educating them about the unique sleep needs of children with special needs and providing them with specialized solutions.

Workshops and Seminars

Regular training sessions led by experts can disseminate practical information.

Online Resources

Easy access to information can be provided by websites, video lessons, and manuals.

Creating Support Systems

Creating a network of support and encouragement can come through building relationships with other parents, carers, and professionals.

Support Groups

Parents can exchange experiences and advice at regular gatherings, either in person or online.

Peer-to-Peer Support

One-on-one interactions with other parents or caregivers who have experienced comparable circumstances might provide insightful knowledge.

Offering Emotional Support

Both the child and the caregiver need to be emotionally healthy. Giving people access to emotional support can reduce stress and advance general health.

Counseling Services

Parents and other caregivers can seek professional therapy to address their worries, annoyances, or feelings of loneliness.

Mindfulness and Relaxation Techniques

Encouragement of stress-reduction techniques like yoga and meditation can be helpful.

Access to Professional Guidance

The best way to guarantee that parents and caregivers are on the same page with the child's overall care plan is to establish regular communication with healthcare professionals, therapists, and educators.

Regular Check-Ins

Regular consultations with experts can help with continuing advice and modifications to sleep techniques.

Access to Specialists

Facilitating access to appropriate professionals such as sleep therapists, occupational therapists, and others for parents and carers.

Providing Practical Tools and Resources

By providing useful tools, sleep techniques can be more easily implemented.

Customized Plans

Customized sleep schedules take family life and the child's unique requirements into account.

Technology and Tools

Advising the use of particular tools or software for tracking and enhancing slumber.

Encouraging Self-Care

It is crucial to remind parents and other caregivers to look after themselves. Encourage regular breaks, pastimes, or other self-care activities to make sure they can keep giving their child the best care possible.

Fostering a Collaborative Approach

A coherent support system is created by encouraging a sense of teamwork among parents, caregivers, and professionals. Trust and cooperation can be developed through regular meetings, transparent communication, and joint decision-making.

Information alone is not enough to support parents and other adults who look after children with special needs. It entails developing an all-encompassing network of support that attends to demands for emotional, intellectual, practical, and cooperative help. These multidimensional support systems can enable parents and careers by offering individualized training and emotional therapy, as well as by creating community ties and promoting self-care.

As a result, the child has a stronger, more resilient support system, which improves not only the quality of their sleep but also the well-being of the entire family. We set the groundwork for a more sympathetic, successful approach to sleep issues by putting the needs and well-being of those who care for children with special needs first.

Resources and Support

Success in putting sleep methods into practice frequently depends on having access to the appropriate tools and continuing assistance.

Educational Resources

Understanding the specific sleep requirements of children with exceptional difficulties and the helpful solutions is essential. Among the educational resources are:

Books and Manuals

Books and manuals that have done their homework and explicitly address sleep issues in children with special needs can be helpful.

Online Courses and Webinars

These offer adaptability and limitless access to professional knowledge.

Workshops and Training

These expert-led courses can provide individualized instruction and practical experience.

Professional Support

Having access to experts who focus on sleep and unique needs can offer priceless individualized advice.

Sleep Specialists

Experts in sleep problems can make diagnoses and offer specific treatment recommendations.

Occupational Therapists

These therapists can offer assistance with sensory problems that might be disruptive to sleep.

Behavioral Therapists

Behavioral therapy specialists can offer tactics for controlling sleep-related habits.

Community Support

Being a part of a group of parents and caregivers who are aware of the particular difficulties can offer emotional support and useful guidance.

Support Groups and Forums

Groups, both online and offline, offer a forum for the exchange of ideas and solutions.

Social Media Communities

Social media platforms can help people connect with one another and create a sense of community.

Technology and Tools

Technology can help track sleep patterns and put measures into place.

Sleep Tracking Devices

These can offer information about sleeping habits and aid in making wise choices.

Apps and Software

Applications that monitor sleep or direct relaxing techniques might be useful tools.

Government and Non-Profit Organizations

Access to services and programs provided by governmental and nonprofit groups may be able to provide funding, direction, and specialized programs.

Financial Assistance Programs

These might assist in providing the therapeutic assistance or tools that are required.

Specialized Programs and Services

Services customized exclusively for children with special needs may be provided by organizations.

Schools and Educational Institutions

By working together with educational institutions, sleep practices can be coordinated with the child's overall care plan.

Special Education Programs

Maintaining continuity in tactics and care can be accomplished by working closely with special education teachers and counselors.

Educational Materials

Materials created especially for special needs education may be provided by or recommended by schools.

There are numerous resources and forms of help available for parents, caregivers, and educators of children with special needs. These resources can give individuals in charge of the well-being of children with special needs more authority. These resources range from expert advice to community connections, technology, and financial help.

We can offer a more thorough and sympathetic system of care by adopting a multidimensional approach that acknowledges the specific issues and provides a variety of support options. It's about developing a cooperative and knowledgeable network that functions as a whole to improve not only sleep but also the general quality of life for children with special needs and those who provide care for them. Access to these tools and ongoing assistance can result in more successful outcomes and a richer life for everyone involved.

8.
IMPROVING SLEEP FOR ADULTS

As adults, we frequently place our obligations to our jobs, our families, and our social lives ahead of getting enough sleep for ourselves. However, to keep both one's physical and mental health in good shape, it is necessary to receive adequate quality sleep.

Assessing Your Sleep Quality

The first step to enhancing general well-being and establishing a good sleep pattern is understanding and analyzing one's sleep quality.

Understanding the Importance of Sleep Quality

Both quantity and quality of sleep are essential. To get a good night's rest, all the necessary sleep stages must be experienced in the correct sequence and for the proper amount of time. It's about getting up feeling rested and staying awake all day. Poor sleep can have a major negative impact on one's physical and mental health, as well as their level of productivity, mood, and general well-being.

Identifying Signs of Poor Sleep Quality

It's important to identify the symptoms of poor sleep quality before moving on to diagnostic techniques. These warnings could include

- Nighttime awakenings that occur frequently
- Difficulty falling asleep
- Lack of energy during the day, fatigue upon awakening, mood changes, and irritation
- Having trouble focusing or remembering

Utilizing Sleep Assessment Tools

The following instruments and techniques can help in determining how well you sleep:

Sleep Diaries

Over the course of a week or two, keeping a thorough sleep diary might yield insightful results. Patterns can be discovered by keeping track of your bedtime, wake-up time, amount of time needed to fall asleep, number of awakenings, and daily emotions and energy levels.

Sleep Questionnaires

Professionals frequently utilize standardized questionnaires to evaluate sleep quality, such as the Pittsburgh Sleep Quality Index (PSQI).

Wearable Sleep Trackers

Smartwatches and other gadgets can track sleep patterns and provide information on their stages, lengths, and interruptions.

Consulting Sleep Professionals

Self-evaluation might not always be sufficient, particularly if the sleep difficulties continue. It is advised to consult sleep experts in such circumstances. They could use:

Polysomnography (Sleep Study)

This study, which is being done in a sleep lab, keeps track of the heart rate, respiration, and numerous physiological processes that take place while a person is sleeping.

Actigraphy

Actigraphy, which involves wearing a device that captures movement, can show long-term patterns of alertness and sleep.

Personalized Consultation

To provide individualized advice, sleep specialists can assess symptoms, lifestyle choices, and other health considerations.

Reflecting on Lifestyle and Environmental Factors

Monitoring sleep patterns is only one aspect of evaluating the quality of sleep. Examining daily schedules, lifestyle decisions, and the sleeping environment are also included. Consider:

Sleep Environment

Evaluating the ambient temperature, noise level, light exposure, and level of comfort in the bedroom.

Diet and Exercise

The quality of your sleep can be considerably influenced by your diet and exercise routine.

Stress and Mental Health

Sleep quality is greatly influenced by emotional health.

Beyond merely counting sleep hours, evaluating sleep quality is an extensive and diverse procedure. Self-reflection, the use of tools, and, if necessary, professional assistance are all required. The objective is to develop a clear image of one's sleeping patterns, identify any problem areas, and take proactive measures to improve.

Adults can improve their sleep and improve their physical health, mental clarity, and overall quality of life by understanding the underlying variables that affect it. A comprehensive and honest evaluation is the first step toward better sleep, and the advantages of this procedure go well beyond the night.

Strategies for Improvement

While acknowledging the problems is crucial, making concrete efforts to solve them can result in a notable improvement in overall sleep quality. Here is a detailed examination of several methods that individuals can use to enhance their sleep.

Creating a Consistent Sleep Routine

The body's internal clock can be trained with the help of a regular and consistent sleep schedule, making it easier to go to sleep and wake up at the same time each day. Weekends are a part of this regularity.

Set Regular Bedtime and Wake-up Time

The body's internal clock is regulated by going to bed and waking up at similar times.

Develop Pre-sleep Rituals

Reading or having a warm bath are examples of soothing activities that can tell the brain it's time to unwind.

Enhancing the Sleep Environment

The setting in which a person sleeps is very important in affecting the quality of their sleep.

Optimize Bedroom Comfort

Maintain a cool bedroom temperature and spend money on a comfy mattress and pillows.

Eliminate Distractions

Make sure the space is calm and dark, and remove all technological devices.

Mindful Eating and Drinking

Before going to bed, what a person eats and drinks can have a big impact on how well they sleep.

Avoid Heavy Meals Before Bedtime

Large, hefty meals might be uncomfortable and interfere with sleep.

Limit Alcohol and Caffeine

These chemicals may prevent the body from achieving deep sleep stages.

Engaging in Regular Exercise

Better sleep is encouraged by exercise, but it must be timed properly.

Exercise Regularly but Not Close to Bedtime

Exercise can improve the quality of sleep, but exercising too soon before bed might be stimulating.

Managing Stress and Anxiety

The quality of sleep is critically influenced by mental health. Among the techniques for reducing stress and anxiety are:

Mindfulness Practices

Deep breathing and meditation are two methods that help relax the mind.

Seek Professional Help if Needed

To handle stress and anxiety, therapists can offer individualized solutions.

Consider Professional Support

It could be necessary to seek expert assistance if sleep issues persist.

Sleep Clinics and Therapists

Based on distinct sleep requirements and patterns, they can provide individualized treatment strategies.

Avoiding Substance Abuse

Sleep remedies sold over the counter can create more issues than they resolve. Always seek advice from a medical professional.

Understanding Individual Needs

Not all tactics are effective for everyone. The best results can be achieved by understanding individual demands and experimenting with various methods.

No one method works for everyone to improve their sleep. To make significant progress, it often takes self-reflection, persistent work, and professional advice. The methods described above offer a thorough method that may be customized to meet the needs and preferences of each person.

Adults can improve their sleep quality by using these techniques, which will boost their general happiness, productivity, and well-being. The goal of improving sleep quality is to improve life in general, not just the night. These methods provide a road map to a more rested and fulfilled existence. Improving sleep is a continual adventure.

How Meditation and Breathing Intertwine

There is a significant and complex relationship between breathing and meditation. Although each of these techniques can be used on its own, when used together, they produce a potent synergy that can greatly improve both mental health and sleep quality. Let's examine the connection between these two methods and how they relate to one another.

The Foundation of Awareness

The concept of awareness underlies both breathing techniques and meditation. Practitioners are prompted to pay attention to their present condition, sentiments, and sensations by this present-moment emphasis, which promotes a closer relationship with oneself.

Breath as an Anchor

The breath acts as an anchor in many meditation techniques, assisting practitioners in maintaining their attention at the moment. Practitioners can more easily notice their thoughts and emotions without becoming sucked into them by focusing on their breathing.

Breathing Techniques in Meditation

To control the breath, clear the mind, and develop inner peace, several breathing exercises are frequently employed in meditation.

Calming the Mind and Body

The objective of both techniques is to relax the body and mind.

They are therefore ideal allies in fostering calmness, lowering tension, and improving the quality of sleep.

Mind-Body Connection

The body's natural relaxation mechanisms can be triggered by conscious breathing control. Similar to how mindfulness and breath awareness techniques in meditation can calm the mind and calm the nervous system.

Synergistic Effect

Combining breathing techniques with meditation can enhance each other's effects, promoting greater relaxation and mental tranquility.

Enhancing Sleep Quality

Meditation and breathing techniques work particularly well together to enhance sleep.

Pre-sleep Rituals

These activities can help to establish a relaxing pre-sleep ritual that gets the body and mind ready for sound sleep.

Addressing Sleep Issues

Insomnia and other sleep-related issues can be successfully treated using techniques like mindful breathing or meditation that are especially suited for sleep.

Personalized Approach

Both breathing exercises and meditation provide a wide range of approaches that may be customized to meet the tastes and needs of each person.

Flexibility and Adaptation

There are many ways to incorporate these practices into daily routines, from deep belly breathing to guided meditation that is focused on the breath.

Accessibility

Both techniques don't need specialized equipment or a lot of training, making them accessible to people of various ages and backgrounds.

Holistic Health Benefits

Meditation and breathing exercises work together to provide comprehensive health advantages that go beyond sleep improvement and apply to other facets of life.

Emotional Well-being

Greater emotional stability and resilience can be attained via regular practice.

Physical Health

Improved breathing techniques and stress reduction can benefit the immune system and overall physical health, including heart health.

The relationship between breathing and meditation is intentional and harmonic, maximizing the benefits of each practice rather than just being a coincidence. Meditation becomes more grounded and efficient and breathing exercises become more conscious and intentional by concentrating on breath control.

This combination produces a powerful toolkit for improving sleep, lowering stress levels, and promoting general well-being. A versatile and effective strategy for health and happiness, breathing exercises and meditation can be used independently or together. These techniques are beneficial for everyone trying to enhance their daily life and increase their sleep because of how straightforward and universal they are.

Common Pitfalls and How to Avoid Them

The route toward better sleep is full of chances for development, but it may also be treacherous. The road to better sleep can be paved with an understanding of these obstacles and strategies for avoiding them.

Expecting Immediate Results

If after adding breathing exercises and meditation, people don't notice a quick improvement in their sleep habits, they could become disheartened.

How to Avoid

Be aware that getting more sleep is frequently a slow process. The key is perseverance and constant practice. Instead of concentrating on immediate outcomes, concentrate on progress and good changes.

Lack of Consistency

Techniques that aren't used consistently can frustrate you and produce less-than-ideal results.

How to Avoid

Establish a program that includes frequent breathing exercises and meditation. Make the routine a non-negotiable component of your daily or nighttime plan and follow it as closely as you can.

Choosing Inappropriate Techniques

Choose breathing or meditation techniques that suit your needs and tastes to avoid disappointment or disengagement.

How to Avoid

Try out various methods to see which one suits you the best. Think about seeking professional advice or utilizing guided resources designed to meet your unique sleep requirements.

Ignoring Underlying Issues

Although they can be effective tools, breathing techniques, and meditation may not address underlying physical or psychological problems that are interfering with sleep.

How to Avoid

If you have trouble sleeping, talk to your doctor to rule out any underlying issues that might need treatment if they continue.

Overemphasis on One Approach

It can be ineffective to rely exclusively on meditation and breathing without taking into account other elements like sleep environment, diet, or lifestyle.

How to Avoid

Take a holistic approach to sleep improvement. Take into account how other elements such as your food, level of activity, screen time, and sleeping environment may be affecting your sleep.

Pressuring Yourself

Stress might increase if you put too much pressure on yourself to "perform" during breathing exercises or meditation.

How to Avoid

Be compassionate and non-judgmental when approaching these practices. Recognize that having ideas and being distracted is common, and then slowly bring your attention back to your practice.

Ignoring the Needs of Children (if applicable)

When procedures intended for adults are used on children without taking into account the specific requirements and phases of development of youngsters.

How to Avoid

When engaging with kids, pick activities and strategies that are appropriate for their stage of development. Make the process enjoyable and involve them.

Using breathing techniques and meditation to improve sleep is a wonderful journey that has many advantages. However, the process may be made more pleasurable and successful by being aware of frequent traps and learning how to avoid them. You can speed up your progress toward improved sleep by establishing reasonable goals, exercising regularly, selecting practical strategies, addressing underlying problems, and taking a compassionate and holistic approach.

Never forget that finding better sleep is a personal and dynamic journey. You'll discover your way to peaceful nights and revitalized days if you embrace it with patience, curiosity, and compassion.

9.
IMPROVING SLEEP FOR CHILDREN

A child's capacity for mental and physical development, as well as their mood, behavior, and ability to learn, are all impacted by the amount of sleep they get. As a parent, you have an important part to play in ensuring that your child forms good sleeping routines for themselves.

Assessing Your Child's Sleep Quality

A crucial first step in spotting potential problems and choosing the best course of action for improvement is evaluating a child's sleep quality. Here's a detailed look at how parents and other adults can gauge how well a child sleeps.

Understanding Sleep Needs by Age

Understanding the specific sleep demands for each age group can be a crucial first step since, as was noted in prior chapters, children's sleep needs evolve as they become older. Let's look at those once more.

Infants (0-3 months)

Need between 14 and 17 hours of sleep every day on average.

Babies (4-11 months)

In most cases, 12 to 15 hours, including breaks, is required.

Toddlers (1-2 years)

Need to sleep 11–14 hours most nights.

Preschoolers (3-5 years)

Usually need 10 to 13 hours.

School-age children (6-13 years)

Usually requires 9 to 11 hours.

Teenagers (14-17 years)

Usually requires 8 to 10 hours.

Knowing these broad recommendations makes it easier to determine whether your child is getting the recommended amount of sleep for their age.

Observing Sleep Patterns and Behavior

Bedtime Routine

Does a regular nighttime routine? A consistent schedule might assist the child in understanding when it's time to unwind.

Falling Asleep

What is the average time it takes for your child to fall asleep? A problem can be revealed if it takes too long.

Night Wakings

Regular nighttime awakenings might indicate a sleep disorder.

Morning Mood

How does your child act when they first wake up? Irritability may indicate restless sleep.

Using a Sleep Diary or Journal

It can be extremely insightful to keep track of your child's sleeping routines and habits over time. Take note of:

- Sleep and waking hours
- Sleep time and the number and length of naps
- Any awakenings or interruptions at night
- Mood and actions throughout the day

Considering Environmental Factors

Analyze the sleeping environment for your child:

- Is the bedroom sleep-friendly (silent, dark, comfortable)?
- Are there any potential annoyances (noise, electronics)?
- Is the temperature in the bedroom appropriate?

Consulting with Professionals if Needed

It can be helpful to seek professional advice from a healthcare provider, sleep expert, or pediatrician if you observe persistent issues or are worried about your child's sleep quality. If necessary, they can perform a more thorough assessment that may include sleep studies.

It takes more than just counting hours of sleep to evaluate your child's quality of sleep. It entails comprehending their age-specific sleep requirements, analyzing their behavior and patterns, recording their sleep, taking environmental factors into account, and, if necessary, obtaining professional advice.

These data will give you a complete picture of your child's sleep health, enabling you to develop individualized plans to promote restful sleep and general well-being. It's important to keep in mind that sleep is essential for your child's growth and well-being, so taking the time to evaluate and improve it can have long-lasting benefits.

Strategies for Improvement

Implementing measures for improvement is the next critical step after a child's sleep quality has been assessed. Here are a few focused and all-encompassing strategies to improve a child's sleep.

Establish a Consistent Sleep Schedule

Try to put the kids to bed and wake them up at the same times every day, including on the weekends. Children thrive on routine. A regular sleep schedule enhances the quality of sleep and assists in regulating the body's internal clock.

Create a Relaxing Bedtime Routine

The youngster can be told it's time to relax by developing peaceful pre-sleep rituals like reading a tale, having a warm bath, or listening to soft music. Here, consistency is essential so that the child understands what to anticipate each evening.

Ensure a Comfortable Sleep Environment

Keep the space at a cool, cozy temperature. Keep the room dark or, if required, use a soft nightlight. Use gentle background music or, if necessary, white noise devices to reduce noise. Make sure the child is at ease in the bed, pillow, and blankets.

Encourage Healthy Sleep Habits

When it's almost time for bed, avoid sugary and caffeinated foods and beverages. At least an hour before night, screen time should be minimized since the blue light from screens can disrupt the production of melatonin, a hormone that controls sleep. Regular daytime activity, but not too soon before bed, can improve sleep.

Teach Self-Soothing Techniques

It can be helpful to educate younger kids on how to calm themselves back to sleep if they wake up throughout the night. This can entail holding a beloved toy close or visualizing a pleasing scenario.

Communicate and Collaborate

Discuss the value of sleep with older kids and work together to develop techniques to make it better. This encourages ownership and raises the probability of success.

Consider Professional Assistance if Needed

Healthcare professionals or sleep experts may need to get involved if your sleep issues are persistent. They can offer specialized therapy programs made to meet the particular needs of the child.

A complex strategy that incorporates consistency, comfort,

healthy routines, communication, and potential professional involvement is required to improve a child's sleep quality. Parents and caregivers can assist their children in getting restorative sleep by identifying the underlying problems and using these techniques.

These initiatives are crucial for the child's general happiness as well as their cognitive growth, emotional control, and physical health. Families lay the groundwork for a happier, more balanced existence for their children by devoting time and effort to improving sleep.

Teaching Kids About Sleep Health

Promoting children's overall well-being requires teaching them the benefits of getting enough sleep. Although it is a topic that is frequently disregarded, it is essential to a child's growth, development, and daily activities. Here is a thorough strategy for teaching kids about the need to get enough sleep:

Start with the Basics: What Is Sleep and Why Do We Need It?

Start by giving a brief but interesting description of what sleep is. To make it relatable, use language that is suitable for the audience's age and perhaps anecdotes or images. Describe why we sleep, highlighting how it enables us to develop, feel well, and perform at our best during the day. The science of sleep, including the need for rest, body restoration, and brain growth, can be explored with older kids.

Introduce the Concept of a Sleep Routine

Talk about the advantages of a nightly routine and how it aids the body in recognizing the need for sleep. Include kids in creating the bedtime ritual and let them select fun activities like reading or coloring.

Talk About Good Sleep Hygiene

Describe the significance of a cozy resting space, such as a cold room, dark drapes, and a comfortable bed. Talk about sleep-promoting habits including avoiding large meals before night, minimizing screen time, and adopting relaxing hobbies.

Discuss Different Sleep Stages

Explain to older children the several stages of sleep, including deep sleep and dreaming, and why each stage is important.

Teach Them to Recognize Sleepiness Signs

Teach kids to notice signs of sleepiness in their bodies, such as yawning, eye rubbing, and fatigue. Describe the effects of sleep deprivation, such as irritability and difficulty concentrating.

Promote the Connection Between Sleep and Health

Stress how getting enough sleep helps the body develop strength and stave off disease. Describe how getting enough sleep affects your mood and ability to concentrate.

Utilize Interactive Learning Tools

Children's books that focus on teaching kids about sleep are available. Make games or exercises that help them remember what they've learned. Some educational applications are specially designed to educate kids on good sleeping habits.

Reinforce and Review

Make the issue of sleep hygiene a regular conversation starter, especially before bed. Reward and praise kids for developing sound sleeping habits.

Teaching kids about sleep hygiene involves more than just telling them when to go to bed; it also involves cultivating a knowledge of why sleep is important. Parents and other caregivers can help children develop a lifelong awareness of the importance of sleep for a healthy life by using engrossing explanations, interactive learning methods, and positive reinforcement. As kids mature and encounter the increasingly rigorous schedules and difficulties of adolescence and adulthood, they will benefit much from this instruction.

Overcoming Common Challenges

Overcoming typical obstacles is a major issue for many parents and caregivers when it comes to helping kids sleep better. Let's explore these issues in greater detail and offer workable solutions.

Bedtime Resistance

Children frequently struggle with bedtime resistance, which can occur for a variety of reasons including worry, discomfort, or a fear of missing out. Establishing a regular nighttime routine that helps the youngster know when to relax is crucial to overcoming this difficulty. Making the procedure more interesting for them by letting them select a bedtime tale or their pajamas. Making nighttime more pleasant can also come from talking to children about how important sleep is and how it supports their development and happiness.

Nightmares and Night Terrors

Both parents and children may find nightmares and night terrors to be extremely upsetting. If it's a night terror, it's crucial to console and reassure the youngster without totally waking him or her up. Talking about your dreams during the day and dealing with any underlying worries may help if they keep happening. A safe environment can be created by maintaining a serene and cozy atmosphere in the bedroom.

Sleep Anxiety

Some kids may experience sleep anxiety, especially if they've experienced scary dreams or are sleeping alone. Encouragement of a comfort object, such as a soft toy, as well as a gradual transfer to their room, providing reassurance along the process, might be useful.

Sleepwalking

Although normally not dangerous, sleepwalking can be unsettling. It is crucial to make sure the child's surroundings are secure and that any staircases are shut off. A healthcare professional may need to be consulted if sleepwalking occurs frequently or is harmful.

Screen Time Before Bed

Screen time before bed can be disruptive because blue light from screens interferes with the generation of melatonin. It can be beneficial to implement a screen time restriction with a cutoff time before night and to encourage alternative relaxing activities like reading.

Inconsistent Sleep Schedules

A child's internal body clock can be thrown off by irregular sleep schedules including sleeping in on the weekends and staying up late. Keeping things on track involves monitoring sleep requirements based on growth and development and maintaining consistency in the sleep routine even on the weekends.

Snoring and Breathing Issues

Breathing problems and snoring could be symptoms of a more serious condition like sleep apnea. It's crucial to keep an eye on snoring patterns and any associated symptoms. If snoring persists, a doctor's appointment should be considered to rule out any underlying medical conditions.

Parents and other caregivers frequently struggle with numerous obstacles when trying to improve their children's sleep. These typical sleep issues can be resolved by comprehending the underlying causes and putting into practice tailored, dependable tactics like open communication, habit reinforcing, comfort and reassurance provision, and safety assurance.

It is crucial to consult with medical professionals as necessary. These strategies can help kids develop sound sleeping patterns that will promote their development and overall well-being throughout their lives.

10. BRINGING IT ALL TOGETHER

In this last chapter, we'll look at how breathing and meditation techniques can complement one another and help families establish a peaceful bedtime routine. This chapter tries to offer a comprehensive plan for putting the methods and strategies covered in the book into reality.

How Breathing and Meditation Work Together

Meditation and breathing techniques work together rather than separately to improve general well-being, particularly in the area of sleep.

Connection to the Present Moment

People who practice breathing exercises must concentrate on their breath, which grounds them in the present. This is enhanced through meditation, which promotes higher states of mindfulness and awareness.

Breath as a Tool

The natural focal point that unites the mind and body is the breath. You can enter a meditative state more quickly by paying attention to your breathing.

Building Awareness

Breath awareness is a common starting point for meditation, which progresses into broader mindfulness and raises general consciousness and mental clarity.

Calming the Mind

Both deep breathing techniques and meditation have a reputation for calming the mind.

Synergistic Effects

They may work well together to lessen the stress, worry, and racing thoughts that frequently keep people from falling asleep.

Holistic Approach

People can develop a holistic relaxation technique that is not only physical but also emotional and mental by mixing breathing and meditation.

Enhancing Sleep Quality

By soothing the nervous system, breathing exercises get the body ready for sleep, while meditation clears the mind.

Integrated Practice

Combining them into a nighttime routine helps enhance relaxation and make the body and mind ready for a rejuvenating sleep.

Creating a Family Sleep Routine

It can be a rewarding experience that encourages healthy sleep patterns for everyone involved to establish a family sleep routine that includes breathing and meditation techniques.

Assess Individual Needs

Family members could have different sleeping habits and needs.

Incorporate Personalization

Make sure the schedule includes activities that are suitable for each participant's degree of comfort, age, and individual sleep needs.

Establish Consistency

The brain receives a signal to relax when a pattern is followed consistently.

Set a Schedule

The body's natural sleep-wake cycle is strengthened by having a set bedtime that includes breathing and meditation exercises.

Create a Supportive Environment

The routine is more effective in a tranquil setting.

Minimize Distractions

Make sure there are no disturbances in the sleeping area, such as loud noises or bright lights.

Include Soothing Elements

A tranquil ambiance can be produced by using soft lighting, soothing hues, or soft music.

Incorporate Family Participation

Collaboration and connection are fostered by engaging in these actions together.

Family Bonding Time

Sharing this time helps strengthen family ties and build trust.

Modeling Healthy Habits

Parents can serve as role models for their kids, establishing healthy routines early on.

All things considered, combining breathing exercises with meditation provides a thorough strategy for improving sleep quality. Parents and other caregivers can establish a welcoming and supportive atmosphere for better sleep by understanding how these techniques work in concert with one another and customizing a family sleep schedule.

This regimen promotes family connectedness, emotional well-being, and long-lasting good behaviors in addition to improving individual sleep patterns. Families can attain restorative sleep and develop together thanks to the synergy of breathing and meditation, as well as careful preparation and implementation.

Monitoring Progress and Making Adjustments

Any successful regimen must include monitoring and assessing results, especially when it comes to sleep. Since no two people are the same, modifications may become necessary as time passes. How to handle this element is as follows:

Keeping Track

A useful technique for sleep management is keeping a journal. Make a note of your nighttime rituals, sleep patterns, wake-up timings, and any disruptions. Parents can keep this record for kids. In addition to manual tracking, a variety of sleep-tracking tools and apps can offer insights into sleep habits and effectiveness.

Review and Analyze

Recognizing patterns and pinpointing areas that may require change is made easier with regular assessment of the sleep journal or data tracking. Open communication about one's wants and experiences when sleeping with family members might promote understanding.

Make Necessary Adjustments

Be willing to try other strategies if one isn't working. Try out different breathing and meditation methods, or alter the sleeping environment. Consult a healthcare provider or a sleep expert for advice if your sleep issues persist.

Celebrate Progress

Every improvement, no matter how minor, should be commended. It promotes devotion to the routine and motivation.

Final Words of Encouragement

Some words of encouragement can inspire people to carry on with this valuable quest when the trip to improve sleep through breathing exercises, meditation, and customized regimens concludes.

Embrace the Journey

Recognize that getting better sleep takes time. Although there may be setbacks, persistence and adaptability are essential. Every action you do to have more restful sleep contributes to your overall well-being.

Family Connection

Use this procedure to encourage stronger ties within the family. By helping one another, the journey can be more satisfying.

Focus on Well-Being

Keep in mind that these routines promote general mental, emotional, and physical wellness as well as better sleep. The benefits of practicing relaxation and mindfulness can extend to other aspects of daily life.

Stay Positive

Maintain a positive outlook and try not to be too hard on your family or yourself. The trip to sleep may be distinct for each person, therefore empathy and comprehension are crucial.

Keep Exploring

Explore and discover more about breathing techniques, meditation, and sleep. Since there are many different approaches, your family may benefit from one of them.

You've Got This

Finally, have faith in your capacity to establish a supportive sleep environment and in the resilience of your family. The techniques and methods you've learned are a good place to start, but your dedication and love for this process will be what makes it truly successful.

The path to improved sleep is paved with connection, growth, and discovery. Families may improve the quality of their sleep as well as their overall well-being by carefully tracking their progress, making any required adjustments, and being encouraged through encouragement.

Despite the route's detours, the result is well worth the effort. You can affect positive change, and so can your family. Sleep comfortably and embrace the journey with an open mind and heart.

SUMMARY

The process of comprehending sleep, investigating various practices like breathing exercises and meditation, concentrating on the requirements of both adults and children, and finally establishing a thorough sleep schedule has been thorough and informative.

We examined the science of sleep, the essential cycles, and the unique sleep requirements of various age groups, illuminating its crucial significance for mental, physical, and emotional well-being.

The discussion included tailored sleep environment improvement options for adults, kids, and those with special needs. We looked at how to spot and get over typical sleep-related obstacles.

These methods have become effective instruments for improving sleep. For both individual practice and family participation, several exercises and routines were given out to help with sleep improvement.

The need to keep an eye on things and persevere was emphasized. Positive reinforcement and encouragement were emphasized as crucial elements in maintaining success.

Emphasizing empathy, understanding, and adaptation, the topic also covered tailored solutions for people with special needs as well as potential pitfalls and how to avoid them.

The emphasis was always on taking a holistic approach and acknowledging the connection between sleep and general well-being rather than viewing sleep as a separate component of life. A path to restorative sleep and improved quality of life has been indicated by persistent themes of personalized care and a supportive home environment.

Enhancing sleep is a worthwhile pursuit that speaks to our core human nature. This guide's knowledge and resources are intended to provide people and families with the power to enthusiastically and resolutely embark on this path. Although there is always more to discover and learn, the stages mentioned here lay a solid foundation.

The relationship between sleep and general health, family relationships, personal development, and well-being is a lovely illustration of how important sleep is. Make use of the methods and ideas described here, interact with the tools at your disposal, and confidently move toward a happier, more restful future. Live well, sleep well!

www.ingramcontent.com/pod-product-compliance
Lightning Source LLC
Chambersburg PA
CBHW070817260726
48660CB00005B/1881